Hostels, Sexuality, and the Apartheid Legacy

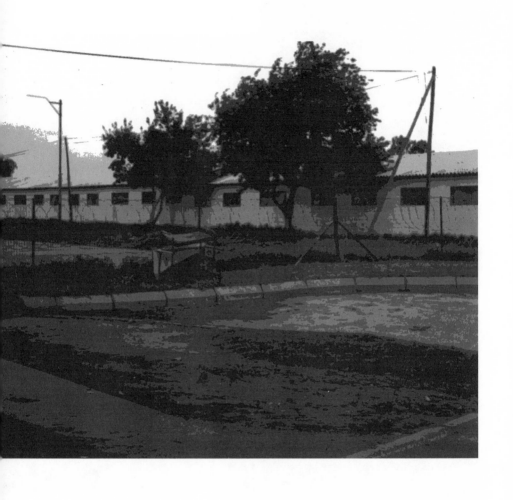

HOSTELS, SEXUALITY, AND THE APARTHEID LEGACY

malevolent geographies

Glen S. Elder

Ohio University Press

Athens, Ohio

Ohio University Press, Athens, Ohio 45701
© 2003 by Ohio University Press
Printed in the United States of America
All rights reserved

Ohio University Press books are printed on acid-free paper ⊗ ™

12 11 10 09 08 07 06 05 04 03   5 4 3 2 1

Maps produced by Northern Cartographics, Burlington, Vermont.

Library of Congress Cataloging-in-Publication Data

Elder, Glen Strauch, 1967-
    Hostels, sexuality, and the apartheid legacy : malevolent geographies / Glen S.
Elder.
       p. cm.
    Includes bibliographical references and index.
    ISBN 0-8214-1491-7 (alk. paper) – ISBN 0-8214-1492-5 (pbk. : alk. paper)
    1. Women, Black—South Africa—Social conditions. 2. Migrant labor—Housing—
South Africa. 3. Lodging-houses—Social aspects—South Africa. 4. Sex role—South
Africa. 5. Spatial behavior—South Africa. 6. South Africa—Social conditions—
1994- I. Title.

HQ1800.5 .E43 2003
305.48'896068—dc21

                                                             2002192674

In loving memory of my sister,

Shona Margaret Elder (1970-2002)

Hamba Gashle!

CONTENTS

ILLUSTRATIONS

PREFACE AND
ACKNOWLEDGMENTS

Hostels, Sexuality, and the Apartheid Legacy: Malevolent Geographies is a hybrid of places and theories. Having emerged in the early morning of the post–Cold War world, the project grew while South Africa was on the brink of change. My intention was to understand and document the changing geographies of a race-riven human landscape transforming into something else. The intellectual project was forged, however, in another place and influenced by that context too. In San Francisco, Los Angeles, Boston, New York, and elsewhere in urban America, lesbians and gay men struggled and organized around an HIV/AIDS crisis. Politics of the body and theories of sexuality, informed by groups like ACT UP and Queer Nation, produced compelling ways of thinking that challenged and invigorated the American academy. Building on feminism, these ideas produced a new paradigm within which to study, learn, reflect, and imagine change. Attempts to blend the geographically disconnected quests for social change and justice in both places inspired and shaped this book. Today in South Africa, tragically, combating HIV infection and overcoming a racist political legacy are seamless geographic projects.

South African geography has been described as empirically applied in method and decidedly averse to critical social theory (as if mutually exclusive!), what has come to be called Queer Theory has been widely critiqued for its über-theoretical, poststructuralist, anti-empiricist tendencies and its turgid writing style. Both projects benefit from cross-fertilization. The study that follows translates sometimes abstract critical social theory and language into relevant South African social inquiry, policy, and proscription. *Hostels, Sexuality* draws from a new theoretical paradigm an insistence to locate sex at the center of inquiry to help us to ask new questions about the South African worlds and landscapes we know.

Ten years later and after a decade of transition and transformation, the human landscape of contemporary South Africa continues to challenge conventional thought, surprise, confound, and generally exhilarate the curious. During that time and not unrelated to interconnecting economic, social, and cultural processes sometimes called globalization, the South Africa context has received an unprecedented level of international attention from world leaders, scholars, students, journalists, and international tourists. Today new AIDS cases are in decline in the United States, Canada, and Western Europe; many people living with the virus in those places are returning to work within the strict confines of sometimes nauseating drug regimes. The HIV virus, however, has emerged with a vengeance in South Africa. Unlike their First World HIV-infected peers, the South Africans who defied apartheid are dying of AIDS, and the next generation of South Africans is born dying of AIDS.

South Africa, a formerly isolated apartheid space, is now integrated into an increasingly globalized network of tourist destinations, knowledge production networks, international-study-abroad experiences, and economic interlinkages. These changes are tangible on South Africa's paved and dusty streets. As present-day nodes of service provision, the mostly former "white only" parts of Johannesburg and Cape Town are a cause celebre, particularly for those who inhabit those now neoliberal, still-pretty white quarters. In other parts of these cities, however, the effects of global processes and connections are less celebrated. Bluntly put, "Early in the 21st century low-income South Africans [will] face an urban existence worse off in many ways than before 1994. Overwhelmed, too, by a 'homegrown' macroeconomic structural adjustment program—including the highest interest rates ever, massive pressure to cut state spending, deregulation, privatization, trade and financial liberalization, and the deindustrialization of large parts of the manufacturing sector—South Africa's cities [will] take an ever greater burden of the pain associated with the growing global economic crisis" (Bond 2000, 363).

The very different but interconnected landscapes of South Africa,

while certainly postapartheid in character, are simultaneously responding
to the heady conditions of contemporary economic globalization. Partly
because of the demands of a globalizing interconnected economic order,
the African National Congress underwent an ideological shift. Perhaps
most visibly, the demands of realpolitik and realökonomie were noted
when the new government backed away from the Reconstruction and
Development Program (RDP) upon which it had campaigned and whole-
heartedly embraced a so called Growth, Employment, and Redistribution
macroeconomic policy (GEAR). Indeed, since it was first publicly announced, GEAR has been highly controversial, and it continues to be so,
particularly among the poor. It is clear through symbolic and real cabinet
reshuffling that instead of the aims of the RDP informing government
policy, economic policy now informs the RDP.

Hugs and kisses resembling something an awkward teenager might
embarrassingly bestow on an old-fashioned aunt at the family picnic are
still reserved for so called old friends like Libya's Qaddafi, Cuba's Castro,
and Palestine's Arafat. Of more symbolic importance, however, are the
South African dignitaries, ministers, and presidents who regularly visited
the White House and 10 Downing Street and have become regular atten-
dees at the World Economic Forum Meetings in Davos and most recently
at the Waldorf-Astoria Hotel in New York.

Days when South African air hung heavy with the pungent smell of
change are now the stuff of popular memory and culture. The long,
snaking lines of South African voters patiently waiting to cast their ballots
in 1994, televised around the world, restored for many living in the world's
oldest democracies a newfound faith in the democratic process. The last
decade has also witnessed, while aghast the world looked on, the findings
of the purportedly secular Truth and Reconciliation Commission presided
over by Archbishop Desmond Tutu in full Anglican regalia: tales and con-
fessions of horrors told by perpetrators, truths told by victims. All revealed
to South Africans and the world that racial intolerance destroys the hu-
manity of those who practice it; truth and knowledge come from those
who have been rendered voiceless. Truth and reconciliation commissions
are now in place in Yugoslavia, Peru, East Timor, Panama, Sierra Leone,
Rwanda, Cambodia, and Bosnia. Indeed, announcing the creation of a
truth commission has become a popular way for newly minted leaders to

show their democratic bona fides and curry favor with the international community (Tepperman 2002).

Like everywhere else in an increasingly connected world, however, South African bodies have also become vulnerable to the human immunodeficiency virus that causes acquired immunodeficiency syndrome. That statement itself has become highly contested within the context of contemporary South Africa. Incontestable, however, is that apartheid's history and its movement-inducing institutions (migrant labor and forced resettlement programs in particular) created a world where people moved around in the past and continue to do so in the present. Coupled with deepening levels of poverty and accordingly challenged immune systems, millions of South African bodies are susceptible to infection by a variety of ills, of which HIV/AIDS is the most noted.

Using a feminist and queer analysis, *Hostels, Sexuality* seeks to chart how we got here. Given that HIV has affected poor women in KwaZulu-Natal most tragically, *Hostels, Sexuality* describes the lives of some of those women during South Africa's transformation. While this study is not about HIV/AIDS per se, the systematic marginalization of poor black women described and analyzed here helps to provide a context within which to understand the spread of HIV/AIDS in South Africa. *Hostels, Sexuality* seeks also to infect conventional understandings of South African historiography, political economy, and geography with a queer, feminist perspective. By locating the politics of sex and gender at the center of an evolving social structure, the analysis aims to shed light on contemporary social policy. While aspects of this latter theoretical approach, informed as it is by feminist analysis and practice, emerged out of the AIDS crisis among gay white men in the United States and Western Europe in the early 1990s, the theories of body, corporeality, and sex are not limited to the politics and bodies of gay white men. *Hostels, Sexuality* is a theoretical questioning and insistence of the need to ask how bodies, sex, and erotics played out in South Africa during apartheid and after. The study also aims to show that bodies, sex, and eroticism are central to everyday social policy. The answers provided are speculative, partial, and intentionally provocative.

South Africans themselves have produced a theory and practice informed by the politics of HIV/AIDS and represented most visibly in the work of the Treatment Action Campaign. That movement's creative blending of the local and global into an antiracist, antisexist, anticlassist, antihomophobic politics in the pursuit of social justice is a profound example South African politics at its best. That work is also firmly located within the proud legacy of struggle that overcame apartheid. With admiration and awe, this study draws inspiration and a sense of urgency from that movement's efforts.

In coming to this point, many people and institutions have provided me with generous support. For funding support I would like to thank the University of Vermont's University Committee on Research and Scholarship as well as the Dean's Fund of the College of Arts and Sciences. Early fieldwork trips for this project were funded by the Organization for Social Science Research in Eastern and Southern Africa, the Clark University Post Graduate Fellowship, and the Mary E. and Irene L. Piper Fellowship at Clark University. To my graduate advisor, Susan Hanson, I am eternally indebted.

For ongoing intellectual stimulation and support, conversations, ideas and suggestions I am grateful to members of the Women's Studies Program at Clark University, Worcester, Massachusetts, the Women's Studies Program and the International Studies Program, both in the College of Arts and Sciences at the University of Vermont, as well as the participants of the North Eastern Workshops on Southern Africa held in Burlington, Vermont, in 1998, 2000, and 2002. Within and outside those United States–, Canada–, and South Africa–based networks, I am grateful to Zackie Achmat, Frank Browning, Michael Dear, Shona Elder, Jody Emel, Cynthia Enloe, Melissa Gilbert, Robert Gordon, Matthew Hannah, Graham Keats, Lawrence Knopp, Patricia McFadden, Heidi Nast, Gordon Pirie, Brad Rink, Esther Rothblum, Richard Russo, Lydia Savage, Joni Seager, Joseph Sherman, Gill Valentine, Beverley Wemple, Jennifer Wolch, and Joseph Won. I am very grateful to Donald Rallis, with whom I taught the South African Field Program in that country in 1995, 1996, 1997, and 1998. His geographer's eye for nuance and change on the transforming South African landscape during those teaching expeditions that he made possible always filled me with enthusiasm and curiosity, making the commitment to this project possible. The views expressed in the book, however, and the mistakes made, are entirely mine.

I am exceptionally grateful to Colin Phurutse, who worked with me as a field assistant in the early stages of this study in 1993 and 1994. His ongoing commitment to this project remains a humbling example of intellectual generosity. I also thank an anonymous reviewer, for helpful suggestions, and Rosemary Jolly at Queen's University, Kingston, Ontario. Her brilliant review of an earlier draft of this work forced me to rethink and strengthen many of the arguments made here.

I owe most to the fluid KwaThema hostel community and to thirty women living in Block A of that hostel between 1993 and 1995. During that time and afterwards, individuals and groups shared insights and life experiences that shaped much of what follows.

Thanks to Gill Berchowitz at Ohio University Press for her support of this project and to Bob Furnish for his discerning work at the copyediting stage.

Finally, thanks to Michael Conley, my partner in crime in some of the United States (but not in South Africa), for his loving support and for his "civilizing" companionship in my new home, the state of Vermont.

The Vermont/Quebec borderlands
Summer 2002

ABBREVIATIONS

AEB   Afrikaner Eenheid Beveeging

ANC   African National Congress

AWB   Afrikaner Weerstand Beveeging

GEAR   Growth, Employment, and Redistribution

IFP   Inkatha Freedom Party

NP   National Party

PWV   Pretoria-Witwatersrand-Vereeniging

RDP   Reconstruction and Development Program

HOSTELS, SEXUALITY, AND THE APARTHEID LEGACY

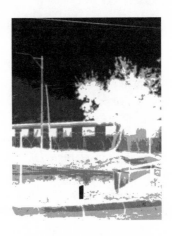

INTRODUCTION
Exorcising the *Tokoloshe*

Transforming the Meaning of Space

THE TOKOLOSHE is a well-known insidious imp in South Africa. He is, according to Zulu myth, a tiny, hairy dwarf who is drawn to women in particular and with malicious intent. In fact, this veld goblin is often described as dragging his oversize penis around, or sitting with it flipped over his shoulder at the roadside, waiting for women. He is known to hide during the day near deep pools of water or in reedy bushveld thickets. The tokoloshe has been in existence since creation. He was relatively harmless until the late twentieth century, when accounts of his misdeeds changed from mischievous to sinister. It is no coincidence that his change of heart appears to have come at the same time the National Party came to power and set about establishing an apartheid order. Recently, then, we should have been expecting the tokoloshe to return to his old, benignly mischievous ways. With the end of apartheid in 1994 surely, like everyone else, he has had a change of heart.

If the evidence presented here is anything to go by, apparently not. Evil intent still stalks the "beloved country." Still targeting women, the apartheid tokoloshe, dragging his phallocentric worldview, is still at work. The phallocentric worldview that seeks to see and organize the world in terms of, or in awe of, the symbolic power of the penis, of course, is not unique to South Africa (for other examples see Bordo 1999). In South Africa, however, more recently the tokoloshe has moved out of the river reeds and is alive and well, living in old apartheid spaces like hostels that used to house apartheid's male labor. Within those walls he continues to frustrate the everyday lives of women in especially cruel ways. While the tokoloshe quite literally featured as a character in several accounts of women who live in hostels, the evil philanderings of the tokoloshe is a useful place for us to start because he is, perhaps, metonymic of the gendered and sexual challenges of contemporary South Africa. During the interviews for this project, some blamed him for sewing the seeds of mistrust between men and women in the hostel community, while others blamed him for the rampant spread of diseases, most notably HIV/AIDS: "Life is hard, and it only gets worse. In this place the tokoloshe makes life hard. We have no money for rent, we have no money for the children's [school] fees, food is scarce, and the illness keeps coming. The tokoloshe is here, in this place."[1]

At a very practical level, it is no coincidence that women living in hostels feel that they are targets of some "otherworldly" force. Since the end of apartheid, and unlike millions of others, their everyday lives have remained the same, or tragically worsened. How does our story change if we see the tokoloshe as an articulation of phallocentrism, or what we will later understand as a heteropatriarchal apartheid policy? What if the tokoloshe is really old policy still hiding in old apartheid's spaces instead of the phantasmagoric creature of folklore?

This examination is not meant to undermine the many positive changes that occurred in South Africa in the 1990s. Rather, the intention of this critique is to assist in reimagining a path toward a more inclusive and tangible Rainbow Nation.

Throughout, I will employ the term *contemporary South Africa*. This is done consciously, to replace the problematic *postapartheid South Africa*, for three reasons. First, *postapartheid South Africa* anchors contemporary South Africa to the past: literally, rhetorically, symbolically, and practically. While the challenges of the apartheid past are deeply embedded in the real and symbolic politics of South Africa and have even found institutional standing (e.g., the Truth and Reconciliation Commission), present-day South Africa is also much more than a shadow of things past. A nuanced analysis must examine the present too; the contemporaneous moment is also bound by broad and deep global economic processes. In other words, contemporary South Africa is like any other "post-something" place, where the challenges of the past are confronted while the challenges of the future simultaneously make themselves felt. Second, the term *postapartheid South Africa* suggests that there is a breakpoint after which everything changes. Yes, 1994 did mark the year that South Africans of all races went to vote for a multiracial government. But what is so often neglected is that 1994 was a *transitional* moment. As the evidence laid out here will show, people live through change in remarkably unremarkable ways. In other words, life goes on for most people in South Africa. The time to look up from the grind of hard work and "celebrate" is a luxury that very few can sustain for long: children need feedings, shelter is seldom guaranteed, dead relatives require decent burials, every morning beds must be made.

The present is senseless without the past but similarly, the present is more than the past. Similar challenges confront those working on "the former Soviet Union," also known as present-day Russia. It is that discomfort that inspires the third reason for using the term *contemporary South Africa*. When South Africa appears without the postapartheid prefix, we cannot but hear the ghost of apartheid chuckling from the other side. In a global context, South Africa is often synonymous with apartheid. Therefore, we augment the proper noun, South Africa, by invoking a complicated coeval present. *Contemporary* is added to this discussion of South Africa because it reminds us to think about that place as layered with time and space.

Contemporary South Africa, then, is a complicated place. There is no denying that the material landscape of apartheid provides the backdrop to our new-millennium tale. In fact, in trying to make sense of change in South Africa we could take Edward Said's advice (1993): one of the ways of examining a country caught up in the throes of change is to examine its spaces. Making sense of change in South Africa today involves examining the transfer of power but, as with all decolonization processes (Said

1993), it also entails a transformation in the meaning of spaces. By examining spaces of change we can begin to unpack the complexities of an apartheid past and an emerging present. Apartheid-designed spaces today, quite literally, represent the dreamy Verwoerdian past under conditions of the present. It is in these spaces that we still find the mean-spirited and sometimes deadly apartheid tokoloshe. One such space is the migrant worker hostel. The ideas, forms, images, and imaginings that inform hostels today provide an illustrative case of spaces under transformation.

Just like the original tokoloshe, who has a history of molesting women, it is no coincidence that the contemporary tokoloshe continues his menacing ways in apartheid's old spaces and especially where women are present. Over the last fifteen years, the "invasion" by women of the pernicious and previously "male-only" black hostel system, on the one hand, suggests a profoundly transgressive spatial act. When women occupy hostel space, after all, the geographies of their daily lives challenge the material, symbolic, and masculine intent of hostels as spaces on the South African landscape. On the other hand and undermining the emancipatory effect of that female invasion, the sexualized discourse that pounced upon the women who tried to live in hostels has confounded their survival strategies. In fact, the tokoloshe may well be the gnarled heteropatriarchal face of apartheid hiding in hostel spaces.

The term *heteropatriarchy* is used throughout to capture the gender-sex system that operated under apartheid and continues to do so in the present. *Heteropatriarchy* more readily captures the gender-sex system than the term used by feminist theorists in South Africa more often: *patriarchy*. *Heteropatriarchy* insists on the ongoing and necessary interlinkages that exist between patriarchal social systems and the politics of a compulsory heterosexuality (Rich 1993). Heteropatriarchy is the social power structure that creates and maintains the heterosexist binary of masculinity and femininity and the associated social expectations (gender performances) determined according to biological sex. Heteropatriarchal constructions represent themselves as the "original" and "correct" form of sexuality and erotic desire, from which all other forms of sexuality have diverged. Heteropatriarchal societies portray heterosexuality as the only approved form of sexual expression. Here heteropatriarchy is viewed as a constituent part of the racial system known as apartheid. This ex-

amination will take place by showing how the outlines of heteropatriarchy are reflected in the contours of apartheid's social geography, or its
heterospatiality.

It is now widely accepted that apartheid was a spatial system of social engineering (see Cohen 1986; Christopher 1994). What remains un-
explained at this point is how the geography of apartheid intersected
with heterosexist oppression. What follows here is an attempt to trace
the sexual oppression of apartheid through the nooks and crannies of
the apartheid landscape. By seeking to examine apartheid policy in this
way, I take for granted the social construction of race and racial categories. While I use the term *race* throughout, I do so with caution. Indeed
much of what follows seeks to show how race moves from the racist
imaginations of policymakers to find material expression on the landscape. It is argued in what follows that one of the building blocks of race
as a social category in apartheid-era South Africa was a sexualized gender division of identity, labor, and space. The heteropatriarchal system of
apartheid was a far-flung and complicated mapping process that divided
the apartheid landscape into what will be described, more accurately, as
a *procreational geography of apartheid.*

Apartheid and Hostels

Throughout the history of apartheid, hostels were quite clearly gendered
spaces. Most obviously, the vast majority of migrant worker hostels were
built to house men only (see fig. 1.1). Although a negotiated, but nevertheless contested, struggle for meanings and identities between male hostel
dwellers and the state took place throughout the apartheid years, it was
only in the mid- to late 1980s that the gendered nature of that struggle
emerged visibly in the form of women occupying hostels. Of course,
"male-only" spaces are gendered, but the gendering of spaces is more
marked when men and women are both visible actors on the landscape.
If nothing else, marking the geographies of men and women helps to
map the gendered differences that existed under apartheid. The gendering of hostel space also reveals the symbolic and actual sexualization of
hostel space—that is, hostels were important to regulate and reproduce a

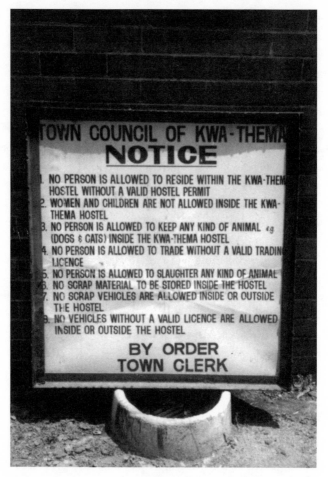

Fig. 1.1. Notice posted at the entrance to the KwaThema hostel for over thirty years. The poster was purposefully removed by hostel dwellers during hostel rioting in late 1990.

certain kind of heterosexuality between men and women. Arguably, we find the heterosexual coding of hostel spaces reflected in legislation pertaining to hostels but also deeply buried in the subconscious imaginings and fantasies of the apartheid-driven South African state. With the occupation of hostels by women, however, the "sexy" aspect of hostel life surfaced, albeit in a different way, in official reports, police records, and newspaper accounts. The presence of women and their sexualized struggle in hostels today simply marks another chapter in what is at least a fifty-year struggle over the meaning of sexed-gendered identities that were constructed, resisted, and policed in those spaces.

While a limited number of "women-only" hostels were also built during apartheid (see Gaitskell 1979), "male-only" hostels are the focus of the extensive, established literature about hostels, and it is that literature and conversation that demands a much-needed gender analysis. Further, this study focuses on hostels that were established by municipalities to house local labor and differed significantly from the more regulated and more widely documented hostels built for gold miners. While hostel life in all forms exhibits commonalties, such as the presence of what Jonathan Crush (1992), borrowing from Michel Foucault, called panoptic surveillance mechanisms, significant differences also exist between different types of hostel accommodation. This study focuses on the sexed and gendered dimension of the smaller-scale municipal hostel.

The sexual foundation and gendered effects of apartheid are among the most important challenges for contemporary South Africa. For example, women make up a majority (56 percent) of the 29.3 percent who are unemployed in South Africa (SAIRR 1997, 359); the rate of sexual crime against women, which was always high under apartheid, has increased by at least 15 percent since the end of apartheid in 1994 (SAIRR 1997, 67). In both cases it is black women who suffer disproportionately, as illustrated by the following account: "Over many years it has changed. I am still traveling around to feed my family. For me, I am struggling more to find shelter. I still rely on my relatives and family to help me. I am an adult woman. I should be independent and strong like my mother. But that is not what I see. What do you see?"[2]

It is no coincidence that while South Africa was internationally synonymous with racism, it was also a site of sex and gender struggles. The contemporary links between racism, gender inequality, and sexual oppression have been well documented in other contexts (hooks 1991; West 1994), but not in contemporary South Africa (for a historical examination of the colonial linkages between race, sex, and gender in South Africa, see McClintock 1995). This study problematizes the notion that apartheid in South Africa was simply a system of racial discrimination and argues instead that the system of racial control was infused with a necessarily

*Cause like
step of not
effect ?*

sexual and therefore gendered dimension that was central to apartheid and is evidently still a problem.

The questions are framed around identity because identity formation is also the site where the politics of the material and representational spheres intersect. Throughout, the material and representational are seldom examined in isolation. Rather, daily life is understood as a negotiation of both elements and takes place in and through space. The evidence presented will show that, while the politics of transformation in South Africa must address material politics, that focus alone cannot adequately redress the material and representational legacy of apartheid.

Representational politics are at the center of the gendered and sexual struggle underway in South Africa. One example of that struggle is its spatial history, found in the complicated relationship that was set up between urban migration regulations that came to be called influx control and the hostel system, designed to house a migrant workforce. In fact the hostel system, which in its present form dates at least from the early 1950s, regulated and exploited both present male and absent female labor. However, the sexual and therefore gendered way in which hostels extracted labor value from both men and women is more often than not neglected by materialist accounts of apartheid. The theoretical (perhaps clinical) debates about migrant laborers oscillating between urban sites of production and rural spaces of reproduction avoids the messy but important ways in which that process was underscored by sexed assumptions. It is the *heteronormative* aspects of those assumptions that occupy our thinking here.

What follows seeks to produce an oppositional discourse to challenge ways of thinking in South Africa, and more broadly. Insisting on heterosexuality's constructedness (by questioning the nature of the relationships it creates between people and places), what follows seeks to illuminate the heteronormative social order embedded in most standardized accounts of South Africa. This implies, throughout the discussion, attention not only to sexuality as an axis of theoretical analysis, but to the insistent pressures of other normalizing regimes pertaining to race, gender, social class, spatialization, citizenship, and the effects of contemporary globalization without losing sight of specific cultural, historical, and local contexts in any particular instance.

Black migration was imagined to be a movement undertaken by

men. The tensions that drew men back to the rural countryside were constructed heteropatriarchal desirings and responsibilities for family and household. Those desirings and responsibilities were rewarded with a virtuous wife held immobile by a draconian state. Thus rendered passive, these women were cast in the imaginings and fantasies of white heteropatriarchal planners and policymakers as the loci of black heteropatriarchal desire and pleasure. A literature about migration in South Africa has seldom granted these "immobilized" women a subjectivity. Therefore, their accounts have not entered into an established system of knowledge about migration in South Africa.

To examine why women remain targets of the tokoloshe (so to speak) and to confront the theoretical conundrum laid out above, I draw on interviews with thirty sometimes migrant women living in the KwaThema hostel, group interviews with hostel and community leaders, and an extensive survey of newspaper articles about hostels in South Africa.

Following this introduction, chapter 2 provides a descriptive account of geographical context of the study. Chapter 3 traces how the successive state understandings of space, evolving sexual mores in South Africa, and an economic stranglehold on "Native" gender relations created a template upon which the racialized economy evolved throughout the twentieth century. A brief survey of colonial, postcolonial, and apartheid law reveals the gendered migration flows that underpinned the apartheid hostel system and how this migratory geography relied on (sometimes flawed but always racist) assumptions about "Native" sex, men, and women. Chapter 4 explores the necessary gendering and subconscious sexualization of hostel space under apartheid. Starting with an examination of the racialized versions of masculinity produced by apartheid, the chapter goes on to explore how homosocial bonding might explain some of the resistance encountered by women who attempt to occupy hostels. Chapter 5 maps and describes the informal reorganization of apartheid's heterospatiality. Spatial arrangements are shown to be the result of balancing competing identities that include mother, wife, sexual partner, laborer, farmer, and informal business operator. Chapter 6 critiques the Goldstone Hostels Report and debates about hostel violence more generally, by way of evidence collected during contemporaneous interviews and newspaper accounts in the early 1990s. It is argued that the geographically marginal "placing" and historical gendering of hostel space ensured that these spaces became the battlefields where patriarchal ethnic struggles for township control took place. Chapter 7 provides an account of the contemporary upgrading of hostels to reveal how the unquestioned sexist assumptions of apartheid embedded in the built environment continue to silence women actors on the urban and rural landscape. Apartheid definitions of legality and illegality, ethnicity, sex, and masculinity and femininity are shown to reify male hostel dwellers' aspirations at the expense of pragmatic and cost-effective (but largely informal) female initiatives already in place. Chapter 8 concludes by arguing that the challenges of apartheid underpin the contemporary health and related social crises in contemporary South Africa.

Gender, Sex, and Apartheid

An emergent and timely debate linking gender, sex, and apartheid has begun to unfold in South Africa, but only very recently. In contemporary South Africa, the new Bill of Rights, for example, protects both gender and sex. The precise meaning of those two terms in that particular context will of course preoccupy the minds of the Constitutional Court justices. For our purposes, I will employ the two terms as follows. Gender is understood to be the dialectical social and political process whereby masculine and feminine identities are constructed from without and negotiated (i.e., resisted, claimed, or mitigated) by those biologically sexed individuals to whom they are assigned. Examples of gender identities include obvious examples like mother and father (social and political meaning) assigned to males and females (biological meaning). In South Africa, however, gendered identities take on added significance because of the many ways that apartheid also created its own repertoire of gendered subjects. For example, rural farm laborer tended to and continues to be gendered as feminine in South Africa. By contrast and despite some of the strongest anti–job discrimination policies in the world, the idea of the urban miners still evokes an image of tensile, masculine labor. By employing a geographical imagination we also note that the spatiality of apartheid meant that many of apartheid's gendered identities were easily mapped in space. In fact, it would not be overstating the case to say that able-bodied black men toiled in South Africa's urban context, while black women labored on the farms and in rural hinterlands. However, the complexities of apartheid come into relief when we attempt to examine not simply how and where those gendered identities are mapped in space— that's the easy part—but what the real symbolic and spatial relationships are between them or how are they mutually constituted—that's the hard part. Put another way, how do we connect the lives of a female who is not only a Zulu mother of four but a sugar cane harvester to a male who lives in the Free State as a migrant miner and who also happens to be the father of her children? In trying to answer these questions we are forced to tackle the sexual assumptions that link their lives because the assigned gender roles that the woman and man take on are not accidental, but rather coincidental in the true meaning of the term. Mother–rural laborer– black woman and father–miner–black man are interdependent identity clusterings that draw on what we might call a procreational worldview. Writing in another context, Michel Foucault suggests, "The family cell . . . made it possible for the main elements of the deployment of sexuality to develop along its two primary dimensions: the husband-wife axis and the parents-children axis. The family, in its contemporary form, must not be understood as a social, economic, and political structure of alliance that excludes or at least restrains sexuality. . . . On the contrary, its role is to anchor sexuality and provide it with a permanent support. It ensures the production of sexuality" (1978, 109).

The interdependence of those procreational and familial identity clusters is based on the roles that the people in question are assigned through biological sex coding. Once coded, the desirings of sexed bodies are directed by the state as well as economic and cultural institutions toward other very specific sexed (and usually racialized) bodies. In turn, we need to consider the consequence of those sexual assumptions.

Sexual assumptions are not the graphic details about people's sex lives per se but rather the ideas that informed the procreational economy of apartheid. By using the term *procreational economy of apartheid,* I mean to imply the many practical and symbolic ways in which South African men and women were and still are expected to father and mother in racially specified ways. It also includes the many ways in which individuals are marginalized when they step outside these procreational roles or choose to perform these roles in places deemed inappropriate by either the apartheid or contemporary South African state. Transgressions might include sexual acts in certain *places,* or sex acts that challenge state-imposed prohibitions against same-gender sex, intergenerational sex, or acts of sexual desire across state-defined race prescriptions. As many of these prohibitions were indeed place specific, a real and mappable pro-creational geography of apartheid is discernible. In other words modern motherhood, fatherhood, and (nuclear, heterosexed) family life insinuate their ways into cultural bodies, places, and imaginings in South Africa: from constructions of normative nuclear familial life and goals, to hetero-patriarchal framings of the nation-states, to the sexualized language used by the police, press, and policymakers to write or explain the world.

Until the links between the political and procreational economy are examined and addressed, transformation will be frustrated by an as yet unhindered procreational economy of apartheid that continues to oper-ate through a pervasive procreational geography in South Africa. As we see in chapters 6, 7, and 8, the policy blind spots occur because policy thinking in South Africa (as is the case in many nation-states) is refracted through a heterosexualized fog. That thinking has frustrated authorities as well as the populations affected in two of the most important theaters of crises in contemporary South Africa: the housing shortage and the HIV/AIDS health crisis.

In South Africa the procreational economy, much like South Africa's political economy, operated and continues to operate in racist ways. Just as analyses of the political economy of apartheid are not necessarily suf-fused with endless details about individual consumer practices, analyses of the procreational economy of apartheid need not include voyeurism. In the same way that the political economy drew on and reinforced racial differences, assigned procreational roles and the expected attendant be-haviors also helped to reinforce the racial classification of particular men and women. Indeed, in precisely the same way as the political economy of apartheid (and its attendant economic geography) relied on but also reinforced a racialized economy and thereby black poverty, so too did the procreational economy (and the procreational geography of apartheid) help to create and sustain racialized poverty in South Africa by defining the terms of black sexuality. Hidden and more insidious, however, the procreational economy of apartheid continues to operate unchecked in contemporary South Africa. The relationships that exist between the woman sugar cane cutter and her miner boyfriend take on added significance because they are no longer economic actors solely but also differently "sexed" subjects in a larger procreational economy (in every sense of the word) living on and moving through an apartheid-inspired, heterosexualized, and therefore procreational geography.

The procreational geography of apartheid is the landscape of apartheid upon which a battery of spatial laws controlled the ebb and flow of South Africa's population. Laws that sought to control urbanization and residential segregation, map and police homeland boundaries, restrict mobility, and so on were unenforceable unless these laws found material expression on the landscape; zones of restriction and enclosure were hallmarks of the apartheid landscape. Accordingly, the geography of apartheid is a telling material legacy of the South African past. Moving through this living ideological museum, however, we can not fail to notice its gendered dimension today. Deeply embedded in that gendered dimension we also find the locales, regions, and places within which men and women were expected to perform the roles set forth for them in the procreational economy of apartheid outlined above. In other words, in seeking to unpack the spaces of apartheid we are also called upon to ask how and to what end those spaces relied on, and reproduced a very particular model of heteropatriarchy.

In South Africa, with very few exceptions, sex as a social category was not spoken about by social scientists at all. Classic exceptions do exist, like the work of Louis Franklin Freed (1949, 1963); however, even these works do not theorize the category sex—it is taken for granted. The brilliant exception to this in the contemporary period is the work of Zackie Achmat (1993), as well as the nascent literature about and by gay and lesbian South Africans under apartheid (see Gevisser and Cameron 1995; Heyns 1998). This oversight during the apartheid era is surprising, given the very explicit ways in which the apartheid state chose to regulate and in fact shape intimate life in that country. In general and at best, sex was imagined, when spoken about, to be located somewhere "out there," in societally marginal places or on bodies deemed heterosexually deviant or deviantly nonheterosexual. In this sense, South African social science

[handwritten margin note: What o heterosexuality is not apartheid inspired. I'm not convinced]

and historiography clearly operates within and reproduces what Butler calls the heterosexual matrix: "that grid of cultural intelligibility through which bodies, genders, and desires are naturalized . . . a hegemonic discursive/epistemic model of gender intelligibility that assumes that for bodies to cohere and make sense there must be a stable sex expressed through a stable gender (masculine expresses male, feminine expresses female) that is oppositionally and hierarchically defined through the compulsory practice of heterosexuality" (1990, 151 n.6). Within that heterosexual matrix, hostels were imagined as being one of those marginal spaces where both deviant heterosex and nonheterosex took place (see Moodie 1994 on same-sex relations between men and Bonner 1990 on female prostitution). In fact, we will see that the procreational geography that marked hostels as deviant served an important role in the broader political economy of apartheid. Accordingly, an understanding of the heterosexual matrix within which debates about hostels operate should inform contemporary hostel conversion programs and an interrogation, more broadly, of all spaces created under apartheid.

As has been argued elsewhere (Crush, Jeeves, and Yudelman 1991; Moodie 1994; Ramphele 1993) and will be taken for granted here, hostels were central to regulating the development of a racial capitalist order in South Africa. Hostels helped to increase rates of profitability by reducing the cost of labor's reproduction. In concert with influx control policies, hostels "absolved" the state, as well as the burgeoning mining and industrial sector, of paying a responsible "family" wage. Instead, heterosexed families were, in theory, housed and sustained in "rural homelands," which they were forced to inhabit under influx control legislation (for examples, see Sansom 1974). Despite the attacks on a heterosexual family pattern through the spatial separation of male workers from families and especially from female family members, the state simultaneously sought to reconfigure a heterosexual, yet altered, black family that suited its political and economic purpose. The state and many analysts failed to understand that other nonheteropatriarchal links nevertheless existed between "rural homelands" and hostel life. Little attention has focused on these linkages or the terms under which they took place, however.

Since the de jure abolition of influx control during the mid-1980s through the "orderly urbanization" policy (and with it the removal of restrictions on the physical movement of black household members), substantial numbers of women have migrated to the urban areas. Some of these women moved into hostels. For many of these migrant women, moving into the hostel was a logical step, albeit one that has been poorly understood by policymakers. A failure on the part of policymakers to understand the movement of women into hostels is evidence of the lack of attention given to the historical links between hostel life and black South African family life. Furthermore, policymakers have failed to recognize that while many women are tied to heteropatriarchal family structures, the actual configurations of lives do not always approximate taken-for-granted heterosexual, or heteronormative, family models.

While most of the women interviewed for this project were maternalized under apartheid, and thereby expected to reproduce the rural black household, their dependency on male breadwinners was seldom realized. Many women, who were also mothers and daughters, lived lives without masculine support whatsoever. There were and are a variety of ways in which women in South Africa live lives within and without the normatized models of family life imagined by the apartheid and contemporary South African states. Indeed, these "abnormal," albeit surviving, women were severely punished.

We can see in the press, policy documents, police reports, state-sponsored commissions of inquiry, but especially within hostel dweller associations, an elevated level of sexual rhetoric about the women who moved into hostels. This all-male chorus was always left unchecked and certainly unremarked upon by anyone. The sometimes shocking sexual accusations against women, unabashedly sexist accounts of sexual violence perpetrated against them, and the blind eye of the state turned toward these gross abuses of human rights beg troubling questions about the deep sexual pathologies that lie buried in South Africa's collective consciousness with respect to hostel spaces. Why, for example, were women hostel dwellers seen as being "at fault" or "asking for it" by living in hostels?

Examining the links between black African women and the migrant worker hostel system in South Africa confronts a fundamental principle of national apartheid: the neat dichotomy between home and work that provided apartheid architects with a national spatial vision of racial segregation. The spatial dichotomy of home and work was also extended to include rural and urban, black and white, and ultimately male and female. By trading a male-centered and economically functional perspective of hostels for a view that examines the hostel as a space, deeply implicated in the heteropatriarchal framings of black families under apartheid, we see that a heteropatriarchal framing of apartheid clarifies our understanding of apartheid hostels not least of all because it provides us with a way in which to see how the hostel was interconnected to and interdependent with other spaces. Further, we are also granted a vision of hostels as sites of resistance. In particular, the movement of women from rural reserves and into hostels comes into sight as a powerful transgressive spatial act that challenges the heteropatriarchal codings of the South African landscape.

The failure by the previous South African government to grasp the complexity of rural-urban household linkages and arrangements as revealed through women's ties to hostel life is possibly one reason why apartheid was never fully effective. The "homeland" system, for example, was premised on the understanding that remittances earned by black, male labor in urban areas would flow back to the rural reserves and support black families. Because the flow of support was unreliable, inconsistent, and quite often only a fraction of the income that was needed to reproduce rural households, women family members were forced to supplement the livelihood of families with earned income as well as their unpaid domestic labor. For women this usually meant flexible and temporary employment that would also allow them to manage their homes. Indeed when women embarked on household strategies to sustain their families and homes, more often than not, those strategies began by rejecting the economic principles of the heteronormative family model (e.g., fathers as breadwinners). That need to supplement income required the unrestricted mobility of women to move in and out of waged labor and formal and informal labor markets. A gender-blind state failed to recognize the importance of women's unrestricted movement in this regard. Myopic sexism that refuses to acknowledge women are subjects is also the reason why local authorities and the newly elected national state are unable to recognize and effectively deal with the recent occupation of hostel space by women, or provide single women with housing. More generally, the current official view also minimizes the importance of women's work to family survival because it incorrectly suggests that only formal waged work undertaken by men secured the material well-being of the household. The official view, therefore, cannot adequately address the consequences of an apartheid past.

Hostels, Women, and Policy

One way to understand the "illegal" occupation of hostels by women is to interpret it as a struggle that revolved around the meaning of space for those who occupy it. A current plan to upgrade hostels by the contemporary South African government is arguably one way to address the housing crisis of apartheid. The conversion of old hostels cannot take place without a reinterpretation of hostel space, however. As women living in hostels have in some ways already contested the "heterosexualized" and masculine nature of hostel space, future public housing initiatives must be cognizant of the feminization of hostel space that is already underway. Not least of all, the invasion of hostels by women and their survival strategies provide clues about possible ways in which nonheteropatriarchal forms of housing might take shape.

Life stories of women hostel dwellers reveal how household struggles for survival in the past were linked to hostel life and remain so at present. Each woman's story was told to me inside the hostel and therefore is part of the clamor of resistance that ultimately overcame apartheid and continues to challenge its legacy. Each embodied life geography must be seen as a voice of survival. Throughout, we note that the interplay of sex and gender created a racialized oppression. Resistance to it is highly significant in shaping the experiences of those interviewed for this project. With that experience emerges an individual identity that is linked to South Africa's history and space.

The primary significance of the information laid out here is in its direct links to the current upgrading and conversions of hostels in South Africa. A failure by authorities to understand the historical context of women and hostels will result in the immediate displacement of literally thousands of other similarly situated women throughout South Africa. These women will be rendered homeless by contemporary authorities because an apartheid-inspired notion of illegality still marginalizes the position of women in hostels. Estimates in the early 1990s put the legal and illegal hostel population in South Africa at 1.5 million (*Finance Week*, 7/30/92–8/5/92). Research based on a Western Cape hostel estimates that between 30 and 40 percent of hostel dwellers are women (Ramphele 1993). To date, a lack of information concerning women's lives in hostels has rendered their poignant stories invisible in the current housing debates and has hidden their ingenious and cost-effective survival strategies from policy planners. Accordingly, the future for women in hostels remains tenuous because of their perceived illegality. Women's status in the hostels is also informed and reinforced by the heteropatriarchal legacy of apartheid. This study explores how a historically imposed racial order was founded on a heteropatriarchal social structure. The differing sexed bodies and related gendered identities and experiences that shaped the so-called racial order of apartheid have serious consequences for equitable planning and policy work in South Africa.

The imperative to examine the heteropatriarchal clutter of the old South Africa is readily seen in the present-day data concerning HIV/AIDS in contemporary South Africa. Tragic and avoidable, it is not surprising that the HIV virus that causes AIDS moves with greatest effect in the population interviewed for this book and in others like it: mobile poor women. Internationally, HIV has infected the rhetorically and politically marginalized and disempowered (Patton 1992). In South Africa, histories of spatial exclusion, forced and voluntary mobility, and laws that continue to imagine women in heterosexualized roles only created a health risk that appears to defy official comprehension. What follows here is one attempt to hear and comprehend.

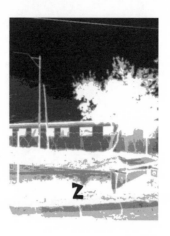

POLITICAL GEOGRAPHIES

IN 1994 the internal political geography of contemporary South Africa changed. Replacing the four independent states, the eight self-governing states, and the four white provincial boundaries, the newly elected government set about creating nine internal provinces (see fig. 2.1). The new South African map has some new regions, names, and boundaries: Gauteng, Mpumalanga. But hints of the old shapes and names dating back to colonial times have also survived: Free State, KwaZulu-Natal (see fig. 2.2). What makes these newer regions quite distinct from the older apartheid-inspired gerrymandering is that they are all contiguous (with one exception)[1] and in most cases approximate feasible economic zones. Masked, however, by present-day maps is the homeland history. As a symbolic first act, newly elected president Nelson Mandela revoked the homeland policy in 1994. Since then, the old homeland ghosts have not found formal recognition, but do nevertheless stalk the overcrowded bushveld squatter settlements and now abandoned elaborate halls of government that were built to assuage the egos of now defrocked homeland presidents.

One way to catch a fleeting glimpse of the homelands' ghostly shapes would be to examine the socioeconomic data that draws lines between

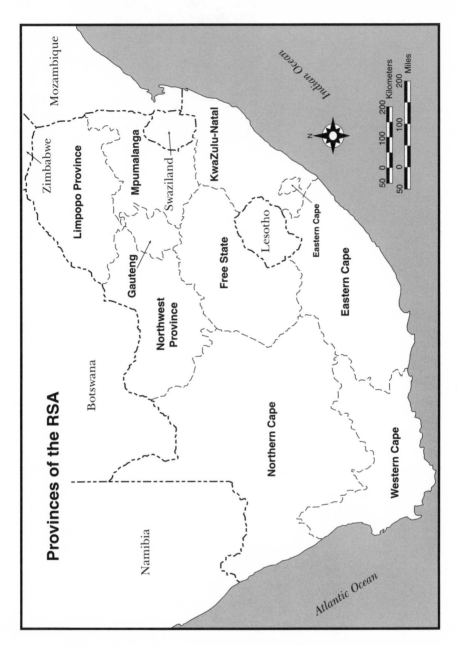

Fig. 2.1. Map showing contemporary internal political boundaries in South Africa

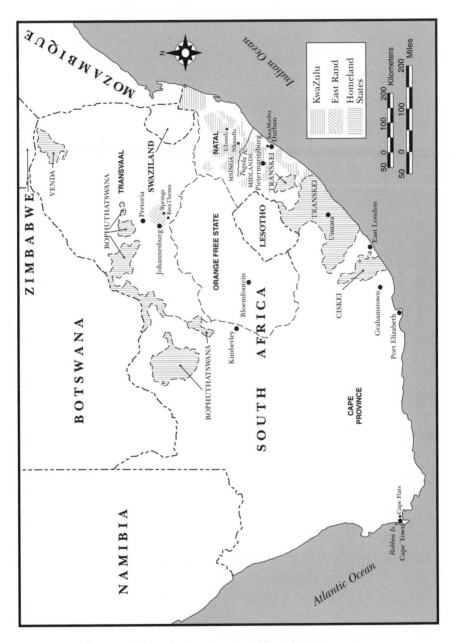

Fig. 2.2. Map showing old homeland and provincial boundaries

South Africa's rural and urban spaces. In some cases, the newer provinces serve as catchment areas for South Africa's most urban centers—Johannesburg and Cape Town. Their respective metropolitan influences are found within the contours of Gauteng and the Western Cape. By contrast, we find KwaZulu-Natal's rural character almost indistinguishable from apartheid's rural homeland, KwaZulu. It is of course no coincidence that new rural provinces, like KwaZulu-Natal, are among the poorest of the provinces. A closer examination of the rural-urban distinctions by way of the 1996 census reveals that some of the largest inequalities exist in the discrepancies between urban and nonurban life circumstances. Of the estimated 31.7 million Africans, 19.8 million live in nonurban areas like Msinga in KwaZulu-Natal, described below. Proportionately more young African children, women, and older people are found in nonurban areas, underscoring once again the gendered geography of apartheid's legacy. The education level of inhabitants tends to be lower in nonurban areas, and income-generating or employment opportunities are fewer. In fact, 53 percent of all unemployed Africans live in rural areas, whereas less than 10 percent of the unemployed white population identified themselves as rural residents (South Africa 1996).

Yet another way to understand the contemporary map of South Africa would be to seek out what other patchwork shapes from apartheid's past, besides the homelands, are still discernible: segregated neighborhoods, impoverished black townships, migrant worker hostels, and so on. Furthermore, what spatial relationships between spaces, configured under apartheid, continue to weave through the landscape? What are the invisible bonds holding places together? Which individuals' life geographies shaped under apartheid still tie space and places together? While new names and places may have given the South African map a new feel, real change is slower. Whether migrants oscillate between the Transvaal and Natal or Gauteng and KwaZulu-Natal is irrelevant if the conditions under which they make those movements do not change.

Here we will seek out those bonds and connections through the politics of heteropatriarchy. Accordingly, we will examine the landscape as a procreational geography upon which individuals move according to the social, economic, and political expectations, demands, and privileges of heteropatriarchal identities (like mother and father). From such a viewpoint, we are able to simultaneously evaluate the extent to which the racialized apartheid landscape was also a gendered landscape. Further, such a vista of contemporary South Africa provides us with a practical viewpoint from which to evaluate or to plot change, or both.

Contextual Connections for Case Study

Within the broader political geography of contemporary South Africa, rural and symbolically female Msinga in KwaZulu-Natal and urban, symbolically male KwaThema in Gauteng are two distinct places and contexts, and as "black spaces" both sites were marginal in the geographic imaginations of apartheid's architects. As a way of reincorporating those spaces into a national South African geographical imagination, the construction of social context in this chapter takes place, primarily, by way of and because of the interlinkages that exist between both places. Places, events, and connections described below are all derivatives of those who live there. These places are documented because hostel residents' experiences of the KwaThema hostel and the Msinga region are closely tied through a myriad of geographical processes that include the economic bonds between places, the construction of social networks, and the subjective understandings of different places that shape experience. The descriptions are not objective. Instead places are sketched in terms that relate directly to the migrant hostel dwellers' experiences. To construct the description in this way, several sources were drawn upon: comments and insights from hostel dwellers, field notes, research diaries, literary accounts, newspaper reports, and personal observations of others in KwaThema and Msinga.

A common theme of violence also ties together the geographies of KwaThema and Msinga. The violence of daily life featured so significantly in the subjective experience of place during interviews that violence is purposefully used to shape much of the sense of place. The description of violent struggles in KwaThema and Msinga is also intended to bring into question the bloodless-revolution thesis that has taken root in some areas of South African historiography. While the scale of bloodshed in South Africa does not rival Bosnia, Rwanda, or more recently Kosovo, it is imperative to examine how South Africa's complex, extremely violent, and murderous recent past shaped places and contexts. If for no other reason, this violent history must be incorporated into any longitudinal study of the headline-grabbing crime wave that "sprang up" in apartheid's wake. A civil war was waged in some parts of South Africa and continues in KwaZulu-Natal today. In this place, apartheid nurtured political and criminal violence.

KwaThema, Gauteng

KwaThema is located in Gauteng, the most economically powerful of South Africa's new provinces. However, even in Gauteng, deep pockets of poverty are sewn onto the landscape. Those pockets are deepest, perhaps, in the string of old apartheid townships that span the sixty or so miles east of Johannesburg. This area, loosely referred to as the East Rand, like the U.S. rust belt, contained (and still does to some extent) most of the heavy industry in South Africa. At a mile above sea level, the entire region is a patchwork of mostly mining-turned-industrial-turned-dormitory towns. Swatches of stark wasteland usually scorched black by winter grass fires separate these towns. Areas that are not charred are so dry that the grass has turned a dirty shade of khaki. Waste piled onto fifty-foot-high flat-topped industrial and mining dumps, usually about a mile long, competes with smoke stacks for the horizon. In her first novel, Nobel laureate Nadine Gordimer describes the drab Gauteng landscape:

> The yellow-ridged hills of sand, thrown up and patted down with the unlovely precision that marked them manufactured unmistakably as a sand castle; the dams of chemical-tinted water, more waste matter brought above ground by man. . . . The wreckage of old motor car parts, rusting tin and burst shoes that littered the bald veld in between. The advertisement hoardings and the growing real-estate schemes, dusty, treeless, putting out barbed-wire fences on which the little brown mossies [swallows] swung and pieces of cloth clung, like some forlorn file that recorded the passing of life in a crude fashion. The patches of towns, with their flat streets, tin-roofed houses, main street and red-faced town hall, "Palace" or "Tivoli" showing year-old films from America. (1953, 97)

Since Gordimer's time, the gold-bearing Witwatersrand of the past and Gauteng of today has undergone at least two, perhaps three, economic shifts. The mines have stripped the earth of its primary deep golden wealth and left on its surface a secondary industrial manufacturing infrastructure. In turn, the contradictions of apartheid and the economy in the 1980s caused a restructuring of compliant capital. This time, plant closures and unemployment rates in excess of 40 percent left the picked-over bones of an industrial base. As a consequence, black blue-collar residents sought work closer to Johannesburg, while white white-collar job seekers found employment in Johannesburg's northern suburbs. In the late 1990s hints of gentrification and revitalization of East Rand towns are reflected in the new brass doorknobs and shiny BMWs found in old middle-class neighborhoods. Young black middle-class families now supplant empty-nested, white middle-class baby boomers. Regardless of race, the middle classes vie for scarce, affordable, and secure housing.

During winter a semipermanent southern-hemispheric high-pressure cell moves in, sealing in the foul and heavy sulfurous vapors that thousands of smelting furnaces produce daily. An otherwise natural clear-blue Gauteng winter sky turns hazy as smudgy dark blotches and rust-colored clouds plume. Most roads across this landscape and between towns are straight and typically deserted for most of the day, the only sound being the moan of an occasional locomotive shunting along the network of railway lines that cut an east-west axis across the region. At sunrise and dusk the chemical fog is at its worst. During these hours the roads and an informal network of dusty paths across the scorched veld are congested with thousands of small black-owned taxi-buses. Especially in the many black townships built by the apartheid regime, gritty and smoked-filled blankets of dusty smoke suffocate everything except the piercing beams of taxi headlights darting across the drab landscape. What the smog does not hide is that apartheid-imposed great distance between home and work, ironically forging a lucrative commuter market for black entrepreneurs (Lemon 1982; Khosa 1998).

Lest we lose sight of the realities of this region, only 64 percent of African households in Gauteng have running water inside the dwelling, as against more than 95 percent of Coloured, Indian, and white households. Altogether, 84 percent African households in Gauteng use electricity as the main energy source for cooking, compared with more than 97 percent of Coloured, Indian, and white households (South Africa 1996). What this means is that every night three-quarters of a million people heat water, cook food, and stay warm by lighting fires in South Africa's most developed province. Of the 3,584,000 economically active persons in Gauteng, 21 percent (750,000 persons) are unemployed. The highest unemployment rate occurs among Africans (29%), the lowest among whites (4%). At dusk, chemical fog and domestic fires compete to fill all lungs with thick and toxic air. Unlike the economic woes of the region, a challenged environmental context affects residents of all races.

Significantly situated on the eastern edge of the Witwatersrand, the township of KwaThema was built to segregate the black labor reserve spatially from the white city of Springs—itself a secondary urban center feeding the regionally powerful Johannesburg. The township of KwaThema was established, seven miles to the southwest of Springs in 1951 to accommodate black families who had been forcibly removed from Payneville (a black settlement situated too close to "white-only" Springs). KwaThema is a product of the strict enforcement of apartheid policies during the early 1950s that sought to enact influx control legislation. In essence the township was built to house an impermanent working black urban population. The exact way in which these urban workers were conceptualized by the South African government is demonstrated by the name given to a suburb of KwaThema: Labore.

It should also be noted that while the establishment of black townships along the Witwatersrand created a visible testament to the "impermanence" of black South Africans in urban area, this process was also complicated by the presence of a small black urban elite. Mia Brandel-Syrier documents, with naive optimism, the rise and complexity of the so-called black Reeftown Elite. Although extremely small in number (but visible), the author was able to conclude, somewhat erroneously, the following about early 1960s life on the Witwatersrand: "The conditions of the time and South African developments favoured their advance. The elite came up in a world desperately in need of them. The increasing industrialization and urbanization of the white population brought, as its natural consequence and prerequisite, the increasing industrialization and urbanization of the black population" (1971, 289). What the author of this account fails to acknowledge is that the fundamental structure of the regional economy was not one that sought to "raise all boats." In fact, white advancement required as its "consequence and prerequisite" the immobilization of women in rural areas and the actual impoverishment of black families, except for a very few. The deepening levels of poverty and simple neglect experienced by towns like KwaThema throughout the 1970s and 1980s belied any sense of social advancement and mobility for all township residents. In fact, the reverse occurred.

Somewhat unreliable figures provided by the South African government in the mid-1980s estimated the population of KwaThema to be 145,500. Of this population it was estimated that 24 percent were women, 33 percent were men, and 43 percent were children under the age of twelve. These figures reveal that the apartheid plan to remove the surplus population of women and children from the urban areas had failed. These data also include 7,482 male hostel dwellers living in KwaThema (Mashabela 1988). The most recent census puts the figure closer to half a million residents within the amorphous, loosely defined, and ever expanding urban area (South Africa 1996).

As is characteristic of all black townships in South Africa, KwaThema is spatially isolated from white Springs by a cordon sanitaire, or an "uninhabited ground designed to prevent the spread of African disease into the white residential suburbs" (Swanson 1977, 388). KwaThema occupies a shallow valley outside Springs, putting it at a physical, visible, and social distance. Having grown up in Springs, Gordimer recollects her childhood with emotive clarity:

> The Town Hall in its geometrical setting of flower beds and frost-bitten lawn and municipal coat-of-arms grown in tight fleshy cactus; the dirty shop-blinds of the main street making a chalky dazzle; the native delivery boys sitting in the gutters, staring at their broken shoes; the buildings like a familiar tune picked out silently on a keyboard: one, one, two-storey, two, one, one-storey. . . . All built of the same dark brick with low tin roofs, small windows and porches enclosed with fine-meshed wire screening which had a tinny dazzle when it was new, but now was tarnished and darkened each entrance with a homely gloom. (1953, 26)

The ordered monotony of Springs (and any other white town in the area, like Nigel, Benoni, Brakpan, or Germiston) is, in part, the result of an inflated white municipal bureaucracy who had, until very recently, at their disposal a cheap black labor force. Both toiled in underemployed boredom to create manicured parks and pavements while black sibling-towns (like KwaThema, Wattville, Tsakane, and Tembisa) lacked basic services like garbage pickup and water-borne sewerage. Throughout most of the region today townships and white towns have been incorporated into polycentric metropolitan areas. Served by a common administration, these metropolitan areas are now responsible for the redistribution and equitable provision of local services. An unenviable task (for an extended discussion of this restructuring and its implications, see MacDonald 1997).

It would not be uncommon to discover that even today most of the white residents of Springs, like white residents in most of South Africa's cities, have little knowledge about the exact site, size, and character of KwaThema. At present, the R22 highway hugs the southern boundary of KwaThema. Until late 1995 the high-speed toll road had no off-ramp to this black township of almost half a million inhabitants. Until 1995, the main access was a secondary road marked by a small signpost at a set of traffic lights. For most of KwaThema's history, this main access road led down a narrow, badly maintained three-mile road, over the R22, to the township of KwaThema. Despite white residents' relative ignorance about KwaThema, the residents of KwaThema are intimately familiar with the city of Springs—both its public streets and private homes. More than twenty years ago, sociologist Jacklyn Cock asked fifty white employers about the lives of their black domestic employees: "When these women were asked what they felt about the difference in living conditions between blacks and whites generally in South Africa, 24 expressed no disquiet. Of these 17 specifically expressed no disquiet, four actually felt anxious to see black living conditions improving" (1980, 166). The relative ignorance and lack of concern white residents of Springs feel for their KwaThema neighbors has not changed that much. Many of the formally employed male residents of KwaThema hold jobs in the large industrial parks, while an estimated 64 percent of KwaThema's employed women residents are domestic workers in the white working- and middle-class residential sub-urbs of Springs (South Africa 1996).

Like many of the black townships on the East Rand, KwaThema has experienced a turbulent past. In 1985 a considerable amount of violence and suspected right-wing vigilante activity wracked the townships. During that period a number of civic organizations emerged, among them the KwaThema Residents' Action Committee, the Thembelitsha Residents' Committee, and the KwaThema Homeseekers' Committee (Mashabela 1988). There is also a strong Congress of South African Trade Union presence in the township, which has proved important in pressuring the local council to build low-cost houses for the poor. An uneasy calm between disgruntled and rent-boycotting residents and an impoverished, ineffective council marked the period between 1986 and 1990. Sporadic rioting and protests continued during this time, while the contradictions of apartheid continued to manifest themselves in other ways as well. Throughout the country, the pressure of economic sanctions fueled the explosive demise of apartheid on a local scale as unemployment rose steadily. KwaThema's informal settlement populations began to increase, spilling out of backyards onto most of the vacant land surrounding the townships. The cordon sanitaire between KwaThema and Springs, however, remained vacant because of a heavy policing by the Springs police force. In the township though, the competition for resources, living space, and jobs in the shrinking Springs labor market became acute.

Between 1985 and 1990 the flow of migrants and refugees from the war-torn Natal midlands reached an unprecedented level. Because Springs is understood by most to be the first major city on the industrial East Rand when traveling from the KwaZulu-Natal plains, it is not surprising that many immigrant refugees sought temporary or permanent accommodation in KwaThema specifically. Because of an acute housing shortage in KwaThema, most migrants moved into the informal settlements or the depopulated hostel. Increasing numbers of Zulu migrants have moved into the hostel over the last decade and the result has been the increasing cultural and economic isolation of this space.

Mahmood Mamdani (1996), Daniel Reed (1994), and Ari Sitas (1996) argue that by 1990 a significant shift in the identity of migrant workers, the majority of whom were hostel dwellers throughout the East Rand, had taken place. A large percentage of new migrants were Zulu-speaking peasants from the KwaZulu homeland. They came from the poorest districts of KwaZulu: Msinga, Nkandla, and Mahlabatini. During the late 1980s a collapsing rural base and political and criminal violence in Natal forced the peasant-class-in-decline to seek work on the industrial East Rand, also known as the highveld.

The growth of the union movement on the East Rand and throughout the country had resulted in an unprecedented wave of strike actions. As industries in the region shifted to accommodate the mobilization of labor, it was widely understood that specific industries in the area expressed a preference for the new Zulu immigrants. A management conference held in the area concluded that "they were hard working, compliant and re-spectful of Whites" (quoted in Reed 1994, 4). This Zulu peasantry was perceived by white employers and black township residents to be politi-cally conservative and reluctant to join strikes and stay-aways. Discipline was entrenched: obedience to the *induna* (headman) was unquestioning. By early 1990 conditions had worsened and tensions between township dwellers and the recent Zulu migrants continued to rise in the township. An unemployment rate of around 70 percent, finite and poorly managed amenities, a shortage of fresh drinking water, and a badly serviced sew-erage system precipitated what can only be called a xenophobic response from longtime KwaThema residents toward the newer Zulu settlers in the region. Sites that immigrants or refugees were known to inhabit were tar-geted. A total of 362 people were murdered in one week of warring be-tween rival groups in the townships of the East Rand (*Citizen,* 8/21/90). Not surprisingly, the hostel and several informal settlements in KwaThema saw particularly bloody clashes.

The hostel in KwaThema was built in 1968 as a temporary urban home for more than seven thousand male migrant workers. Mounting pressure in the township, augmented by the fact that increasing numbers of Zulus had moved into the hostel, reached a breaking point in August 1990:

> In KwaThema on the East Rand yesterday afternoon, thousands of young township residents surrounded burnt-out hostels in which it was alleged that certain Zulu elements were held up with AK-47 assault rifles. Earlier the bodies of seven hostel dwellers were shown to reporters. Some of the victims had apparently been shot by AK-47s, some had been hacked to pieces and others were castrated. . . .
>
> Hostel residents were seen streaming out of the township with their possessions, in a bid to escape the escalating violence. . . . The violence between primarily Zulu hostel dwellers and other township residents,

many of whom support the African National Congress also resulted in the hostel being set alight. (*Citizen*, 8/21/90)

The graphic account relies on the spatial categorization of individuals and the implicit causality that labels like "primarily Zulu" and "many of whom support the African National Congress" create. The patriarchal, masculine, and phallic nature of this description elides the fact that at this time there was a female presence living in the hostel. The tension between Zulu migrants and long-term KwaThema residents as represented in local township politics and mythology, the media, and national politics still echoes in contemporary South Africa. Today, an ethnopolitical analysis of South Africa or its hostel system is commonplace. It is worth remembering, however, that these arguments came into popular vogue only as recently as the late 1980s and early 1990s. Before that time "ethnic" arguments were very often seen as part of an apartheid-inspired ideology. Even in the early 1990s, all reports were not presented in the same terms. The quote above, which was taken from the conservative Nationalist government–supported *Citizen* newspaper is different from the story about the KwaThema events in the *Sowetan* (a newspaper with a predominantly urban black readership):

> More than 1000 militant youths toyi-toyied[2] and milled around the burning hostel, trapping hundreds of hostel dwellers inside for a long period. The youths said they had come to support hostel dwellers, not to become involved in the fight. They "also wanted to see the hostel down [destroyed]." . . .
>
> Groups of people armed with hammers attacked the walls of the burning buildings before police stopped them. Hundreds of dwellers left the besieged hostel as police escorted others to collect their possessions. (*Sowetan*, 8/21/90)

The generational categories used by the *Sowetan* and the ethnopolitical labels employed by the *Citizen* serve to underscore the complexity of the identity of those associated with the KwaThema hostel. The *Sowetan* distinguishes between the young township residents and the hostel by focusing on the attempt by attackers to dismantle the hostel. A week later the *City Press* (a Johannesburg-based black urban newspaper) reported: "ANC aligned organizations will hold a mass meeting in

KwaThema, Springs, today to discuss the thorny issue of their removal of hostels from the area. Hostel dwellers have had little sleep as a result of running battles with Zulu impis [traditional term used to describe Zulu warrior] in the saga of violence which has left more that 500 dead" (*City Press*, 8/26/90).

Protracted news coverage constructed the hostel dwellers and their attendant "impi" regiments as "the problem" in KwaThema. Accordingly, the debate at a township and national level moved away from the material injustices that had led to the violence. Instead political leaders and the press implicitly supported a representation of Zulu masculinity as violent.

Almost two years later and after an increased level of public discourse around ethnicity as the root of the violence in South African's townships, it was reported that, "in spite of outraged cries of No from residents, the notorious single men's hostel in KwaThema will soon be removed" (*City Press*, 6/7/92). This time the violence of two years ago was described in ethnolinguistic terms as a pitched battle within the hostel between "Xhosa-speaking migrant workers" who were driven out of the hostel by "heavily armed IFP [Inkatha Freedom Party] impis." The same report stated that an agreement to renovate the hostel had been set in place. The plan was to renovate the burned-out buildings and turn sections into family units (*City Press*, 6/7/92).

Throughout the mid 1990s, people inhabited the hostel. An uneasy and at times violent accord was set in place between long-term township residents and hostel dwellers, usually identified as Zulus. Superficial repairs to the hostel have rendered it somewhat livable. Burned-out buildings are now painted, and council-provided roofing and windows protect some seven hundred residents from the elements. Despite the uneasy truce in place, the hostel in KwaThema remains a contested space. Tension is evident on the physical landscape and in the imaginings of the hostel residents inside its barbed-wire fence and the residents in the neighboring township. The hostel has assumed an almost mythical dimension in the popular imagination of township residents. One township woman remarked, "They practice magic and cast spells on the township from inside the hostel. The violence will end only when they [the Zulu hostel dwellers] leave, and the hostel is removed."[3]

Most of the hostel infrastructure was destroyed by fire during a riot in September 1990. Between 1991 and 1995 approximately two thousand "bed spaces" were inhabitable. According to hostel records in 1993, approximately eight hundred residents paid twelve rands ($1.50) per month for hostel space. The hostel manager, however, estimated that approximately two thousand were actually living in the hostel.[4]

Inside the hostel lives a community under siege. Because men and women hostel dwellers find themselves living at odds with many in their surrounding community, they are often scared to venture outside the hostel boundaries. Clearly this is not the case with all hostel dwellers, especially those who have a personal history in KwaThema that extends beyond the violence of 1990. Even those who manage to move between both spaces, however, do so at personal risk: "I am tired of people pointing fingers at me, even my own family saying, She is a Zulu from the hostel. . . . so now I try to keep inside the hostel as much as possible."[5]

Living within these emotional and real boundaries, residents have sought self-sufficiency. A herd of cattle and crops of maize and millet compete for space inside the crowded compound, under the constant surveillance of a cowherd and an armed personnel carrier. The armed police, however, maintain a watchful presence.

The yards between hostel rooms are sites of constant activity during the day. Muddy and littered, the outdoor spaces are also filled with noise. The blaring of a radio from the spaza shop (a small informal grocery store) set up by one of the female hostel residents competed with the conversations of ten or more women tending fifty-gallon drums of beer brewing on open fires. Unemployed or shift-work men seeking to buy beer drift in and out of the area. Some stay a while, other men leave a trail of beer as they carry leaky buckets back to their rooms in other sections of the hostel. At night the sounds of Dolly Parton, Sipho "Hotsticks" Mbuza, Brenda Fassi, and hostel conversations give way to an eerie silence broken by the occasional rattling of gunfire or screeching of car tires.

Inside the actual buildings that encircle the open spaces, hostel dwellers have gone to considerable effort to create a livable space. All rooms in KwaThema were originally designed to house twenty workers on concrete bunks. By removing some of these bunks, many women hostel dwellers have reclaimed the concrete floors and unventilated rooms as family living spaces and beer breweries. Magazine pictures of Magic Johnson, Iwisa Kaizer Chiefs (a historically Zulu-supported soccer team), Mangosuthu Buthelezi, and the Zulu monarch King Goodwill Zwelithini in happier times, and an advertisement for shoes peer down from the rough cast plaster walls. Alternatively, the familiar red, green, and yellow colors and IFP letters are emblazoned on the walls. Most residents in this section of the hostel are women, and they have created personal living spaces by hanging sheets, or in one case, by building a lockable door into a wooden wall. Blurring any simplistic division of space, sleeping areas are also storage space for beer-brewing supplies.

More recently, rebuilding the hostel and converting these contested spaces into family housing has meant that a parallel set of lives has been added to the hostel environment. Contractors, builders, planners, and new families have begun to move through and occupy recently renovated spaces.

Msinga, KwaZulu-Natal

At a first glance, the precise circumstances and material realities of the KwaThema hostel stand in stark contrast to Msinga, some three hundred miles to the southeast, where most of the KwaThema hostel dwellers originated. Here in the present-day KwaZulu-Natal midlands, washed by maritime winds depositing rains as they ascend the Drakensberg Mountains, particles of the former KwaZulu homeland region are sprinkled. During the 1980s KwaZulu refused to accept the independence that was foisted upon other "homelands" in South Africa. Unlike Bophuthatswana, Ciskei, Transkei, and Venda, all of whom "endured" independence, KwaZulu accepted a regional form of administrative power instead. In return for the divestment of responsibility, the South African government rewarded KwaZulu leaders (Buthelezi and the regional Zulu monarch, Zwelithini) with an infrastructure at Ulundi and a yearly operating budget in excess of $3.5 million (SARB 1991). In a spirit of compromise today, both Pietermaritzburg, the former capital of Natal, and Ulundi are alternating administrative capitals of KwaZulu-Natal. In delineating the boundaries of KwaZulu, the white South African government was able to gerrymander lines around the informal settlements encircling Natal's "white" cities—Durban and Pietermaritzburg. Lines around the informal suburbs of Edendale in Pietermaritzburg and KwaMashu in Durban made it possible for the South African government to ignore the urban housing demands of citizens. By reconstructing the identity of Edendale and KwaMashu residents into that of rural KwaZulu nationals, these "reconstituted" urbanites were also denied access to the regional tax base they contributed to through income tax on urban jobs and a 14 percent sales tax on purchases bought in Durban or Pietermaritzburg. Today, and because of an abolished homeland system, Durban and KwaMashu are once again related spaces on the South African urban landscape. Called the Durban Metro Council, council members from white Durban and black KwaMashu work alongside six other local councils to provide a comprehensive range of regional urban services.

The former KwaZulu was made up of nine geographic parcels of state-allocated land that have precipitated a local and very sensitive political climate throughout present-day KwaZulu-Natal. The 1999 elections revealed that KwaZulu-Natal remains a highly contested and deeply divided political terrain. It was the residents of KwaZulu-Natal that stood in the way of the African National Congress attaining a two-thirds majority in the National House of Assembly in 1999. In fact, by a slim margin (40.45% to 39.78%), the Zulu nationalist Inkatha Freedom Party held onto regional power in KwaZulu-Natal in 1999. More so than anywhere else, these most recent election results attest to how the fractious local politics fermented under apartheid continue to seethe today.

The borders of the former homeland spaces also abut and encroach upon other local communities, physically and culturally. More than a simple contestation of physical borders, the geography of apartheid bequeathed a low-grade, context-driven cultural war. Perhaps one of the more racialized examples is found in a crescent stretching through northern and eastern KwaZulu-Natal. It is along this half-moon that the former KwaZulu border at different points nudged, incorporated, and threatened the conservative white Afrikaans-speaking heartland. The perceived threat experienced by conservative Afrikaners might explain the now waning support enjoyed by the paramilitary, neo-Nazi Afrikaner Resistance Movement (Afrikaner Weerstand Beweeging, AWB) in that area. Because close to 76 percent of KwaZulu-Natal is rural and a large portion of the arable land has been farmed by Dutch trekboer settlers since the Zulu wars of the mid-1800s, stretches of KwaZulu-Natal mark the symbolic contested terrain of a late-twentieth-century struggle between Zulus and Boers.

That contest has occurred among administrators and has been fought at the community level by rural terrorists on both sides. More recently, however, and using the most recent election results as a bellwether, both the former ruling National Party and the newly formed Afrikaner Eenheid Beweeging (AEB, Afrikaner Unity Movement) suffered humiliating defeats throughout the area. Perhaps, this defeat was no more symbolic than in the small town of Vryheid, where the Zulu-dominated IFP attained 52 percent of the vote and the AEB managed a meager 0.3 percent. The decimation of Afrikaner influence in Vryheid takes on added significance because of its close proximity to the hallowed Blood River battle site, where Afrikaner myth making claims a holy alliance between God and the trekboers gave them a miraculous victory over the formidable Zulu warriors in 1838 and a manifest destiny to rule South Africa.

The 1996 census reflected that, like the figures in 1990, KwaZulu has the highest ratio of persons-per-hectare to arable land in the country (South Africa 1990, 1996). Demographers need look no further than the heavily eroded hillsides, deep ditches, and silted tributaries that scratch the historically fertile and lush valleys to realize that KwaZulu is overpopulated and has been for more than sixty years (Wilson and Ramphele 1989).

As mentioned before, African households in nonurban areas are unlikely to have access to electricity, running water, flush toilets, or telephones. Fetching wood and carrying water are important nonurban life-sustaining activities. In fact, only 7.5 percent of African households in nonurban areas in KwaZulu-Natal have running water inside their homes, a mere 14 percent use electricity as the main energy source for cooking, and only 2.7 percent have a land-line telephone in the dwelling.

Unemployment in the country remains high (29 percent), but slightly lower than 1994 (33 percent). However, this definition of unemployment does not take into account how people sustain themselves and their households. In KwaZulu-Natal, as in Gauteng, work is not necessarily waged work, and householders may be involved in such activities as subsistence agriculture, exchange of goods and services, or fuel gathering, all of which are unpaid activities. However, of the 2,724,000 economically active persons in KwaZulu-Natal 33 percent (901,000 persons) are unemployed. The highest unemployment rate occurs among Africans, namely 30 percent (829,000 persons). For Coloureds the unemployment rate is 18.2 percent, for Indians it is 14.2, and for whites 5.8 (South Africa 1996).

Unlike KwaThema, rush hour in the Tugela Ferry area in KwaZulu-Natal is a gaggle of thirty uniformed schoolchildren walking down the long, straight dirt road that plunges into one of the deepest valleys in the region. A lone single taxi races by, raising a cloud of dry, red dust. The group gets smaller as the children peel off toward their homes scattered throughout the hills. Then there is silence again and nothing moves except for the grating gears of the state-sponsored (some might suggest occupying) South African Security Services jeep as it moves noisily some distance away. The irony of this "peace-keeping" deployment escapes no one.[6]

The central valley of KwaZulu-Natal, the region known as Msinga to locals, flanks the Tugela River. The encircling mountain walls that during earlier times trapped life-giving rains over the valley now trap inhabitants in an ecological wasteland. Peaks and hilltops look down on the valley. Their ancient names suggest that life has never been easy in these parts: Sikhaleni (the reason for crying), Kwamathonsi (the place of little water or madness). Echoes of sadness inflect the opening to *Cry, the Beloved Country* as Alan Paton uses a nearby landscape to open his tragic novel:

> The great red hills stand desolate, and the earth has torn away like flesh. The lightning flashes over them, the clouds pour down upon them, the dead streams come to life, full of the red blood of the earth. Down in the valleys women scratch the soil that is left, and the maize hardly reaches the height of a man. They are valleys of old men and women, of mothers and children. The men are away, the young men and girls are away. The soil cannot keep them anymore. (1950, 4)

Paton's attention to both the environmental and gendered effects of apartheid should not escape the curious reader. Stripped of topsoil and men, the Ixopo valley lies wasted and vulnerable, in Paton's view. Although the reality was somewhat more complicated, today inland KwaZulu-Natal shows a landscape compounded by the intervening apartheid years.

During the hot summer months, the orographic local climate brings in ink-blue, anvil-shaped cumulonimbus clouds that drench the valleys. The resulting thunderstorms that drum-roll through the central valleys of KwaZulu-Natal in the late afternoons of summer result in torrrential downpours as deadly as an acid wash. The intense towering storms dwarf the overcultivated valleys and the impoverished population. Storms lash away at the precious thin film of soil covering the valley. Following downpours, there is the sound of running water and the sight of fragile, flimsy-rooted crops, torn from their shallow soil beds, awash in a stream of mud and garbage. Bound for the Indian Ocean, the eastward-flowing Tugela River whisks away promise and sustainability. Left behind is a scoured-out, hard, and withered countryside.

As a visitor approaches the homesteads in places like Tugela Ferry, the close link between life and death takes on a geographical twist. Alongside the white painted homestead are graves. The macabre scene is repeated over and over throughout the area. Even in death, these rural inhabitants compete for space. In between maize plants, graves of various sizes and age reveal at once the morbid details of a violated community for whom grieving the loss of children, parents, and friends has become a way of life.

Graves too tell stories here. Memorial stones from eighty years ago tell of a time when old age and death were sojourners. More recent hastily constructed wooden crosses tell of lives ended too quickly. A fifteen-year-old boy lies close to his sixty-seven-year-old grandfather. Since the mid-1990s, the human immunodeficiency virus that causes AIDS (a view not taken for granted in these parts) has stalked the region. Now it is it impossible to tell whether death has come to the young through violence or disease. A barbed-wire fence keeps the goats out of the rapidly expanding burial ground. As an added precaution, the six, eight, or (in one case) fifteen mounds are covered with dead thorn bushes. The stillness becomes oppressive. A half mile along the road at another kraal, the dogs lie in the humid sun, chickens scratch, and in a flash of déjà vu Dolly Parton again blares out the windows. Like the noisy hostel room, this home is a she-been, or illicit brewery and speakeasy. An ambushed small truck sits in the yard with six bullet holes in the windshield. Next to it is a burned-out car riddled with the familiar neat, round punctures. Men in overalls loll on benches around two circular thatched huts. The huts are of the traditional design, with white walls and thickly matted rush roofs. Once again, deathly mounds of red soil mock the rural idyll. Inside the small homestead it is cool, with a large, clear floor space. Rolled sleeping mats and stacked boxes furnish this particular home. Inside these walls a living space is also a common area for the preparation of ingredients for beer brewing, which the female members of the household perform.

The stranglehold of violence that has laid claim to this part of South Africa during the last century and a half must inform any contemporary analysis of those who live on its political knife-edge. Most recent data suggest that things are not improving. When compared to the other eight provinces in South Africa, KwaZulu-Natal held either first or second place in national rates of attacks on the elderly (29 percent), attacks on farms and smallholdings (20 percent), murders (28 percent), and rapes (17 percent). No other province appears with the frequency of KwaZulu-Natal in overall crime statistics. In a region often understood to be a gerontocracy, attacks on the elderly are particularly revealing and troubling. And, while the precise reasons for the high level of crimes are debated and anchored in the past, present, and future, there is no disagreement that the figures evince a deeply wounded community.

Political Geography, Power, and Place

The above descriptions have drawn out some of the mutually constituted ways in which "places" exist in the imaginings of those who live in and between them. Emphasis was given to the KwaThema hostel because it is the focus of the study. While the descriptions have shown the context-specific way in which apartheid was experienced, Msinga and the hostel in KwaThema are also enmeshed in a series of wider events. Their inclusion in this study serves as background to the analysis that follows.

One way of understanding the relationships between these two places is to locate both as nodes on the procreational geography of apartheid. The similarities and differences described above are interesting because they reveal to us how the demands of the procreational economy of apartheid were crafted and resisted in specific places. Domestic rural spaces and public urban spaces were never independent locales in the minds of those who moved between them. Experiences of place and the connections that bind them are at the core of understanding migration in South Africa, and especially under apartheid, because migration was a system premised on the divisions of space. When we seek out those connections from a gendered and sexed perspective, the lives of men and women and how they related to each other are easier to discern.

Environmental damage and political violence are two examples of how apartheid has affected both places. KwaThema and Msinga are place-specific scars on the landscape of contemporary South Africa. They are also sites of remembrance, places of struggle, and home to working people who negotiate spatial tensions between them in order to live.

Doreen Massey argues that traditional arguments about place have suggested an essential identity contained within distinct boundaries: "Conceptualizing space, mobility and access in a more socially imaginative way, and abandoning an easy and excited notion of generalized and undifferentiated time-space compression, might enable us to confront some of these issues more inventively" (1993, 36). Her challenge reverberates within this study, which seeks to move beyond a static notion of identity. Msinga and the KwaThema hostel are independent places on the South African map, but for the residents of the hostel they are intimately defined by their linkages through time and space and as such provide opportunities for survival.

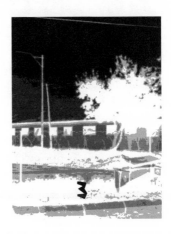

APARTHEID FANTASIES

> In constructing a notion of differentiated citizenship . . .
> the gendering of citizens is a topic too often ignored. . . .
> If citizens were to be properly controlled, the family was
> a key modal unit through which this control was to be ex-
> ercised and proper citizens . . . were to be created. Houses
> were built (if inadequately) for families, and only families
> could inhabit them. Women were persistently conceived of
> as "housewives" by administrators in a community where
> women were frequently breadwinners, even if through in-
> formal work rather than formal employment. . . . That
> the administrators were all men is perhaps unsurprising.
> But that image of fatherhood, and the punitive character-
> istics of this social and familial role, were central to the
> exercise of power in locations is a direct consequence of
> the masculine character of the state. As with questions of
> racialized political identity, the gendered character of
> apartheid state power requires a lot more research.
>
> —Jennifer Robinson, *The Power of Apartheid*

IT IS SURPRISING, as Robinson suggests, that the gendering of apartheid has not received more attention. Instead, what has been documented
are the ways that men sought to dominate each other, or more recently,

how undifferentiated gendered subjects resisted domination. Exceptional works by Belinda Bozzoli (1991) and Julia Wells (1993) suggest that the undifferentiated subjects in most accounts were men, but men were part of families. In those families, women worked to "reproduce labor" in theory and practice.

In what is hopefully an obvious point, I add to Robinson's insights by arguing that the family within which women's experiences were cast was not just any family; the family of apartheid theory is a heterosexual family and in order to understand how gender operated in South Africa and during apartheid, we must ask these questions in the context of the procreational economy of apartheid. In other words, how and to what end was family life in South Africa assumed to follow a particular heterosexual norm? Furthermore, how do we interpret acts by individuals who chose to resist the imposition of a particular vision of heteropatriarchy?

Consider for a moment the possibility that not all women living in rural southern Africa desire men (or wish to marry men and by way of heterosexual sex reproduce children). Indeed, for over two decades it has been argued that "woman-woman marriage—in which one woman pays brideprice to acquire a husband's right to another woman—has been documented in more than thirty African populations, including at least nine Bantu-speaking groups in present-day southern Africa" (O'Brien 1977; quoted in Carrier and Murray 1998, 255). While it helps little to overstate the degree to which same-sex desire shapes desire in southern Africa, the possibility should not be ignored. Indeed, it is also important to see nonnormative heterosexual politics as part of the political struggle that finally overcame apartheid (see Gevisser and Cameron 1995). However, even within this nascent literature, and certainly southern African historiography more generally, rural female same-sex support and desire is all but ignored. The documented erotic relationships among Basotho women in Lesotho, documented by Kendall (1998), stands out as an exception. Conclusions such as hers, that "love between women is as native to southern Africa as the soil itself" (224), are rare and my intention is more modest than to document same-sex erotics. Consider how things change, however, if we locate these findings alongside those of Andrew Spiegel (1991), seeking to demythologize heterosexual "polygyny" in Lesotho. By rejecting the dictates of the heterosexual matrix, we can begin to ask whether and when women's sexual extramarital relations do not include men but rather other women? What I am seeking to show is how a particular vision of heterosexuality underscored both policies that shaped migrant life in South Africa, as well as the theories that sought to understand that process.

It is also difficult to conduct such an analysis without also asking why South African historiography, more generally, has operated within an unquestioned heterosexual maze of meaning. However, the latter critique is one that will be further examined in the following chapter. Here we will see how distinctly gendered life geographies were wrought by an apartheid state seeking to inscribe, through fantasy and policy, a particular vision of heterosexuality that would be marked in space and time. By rendering a view of the landscape in this way, it will become evident that the state's heterosexual visioning created a real landscape in apartheid South Africa and not simply a symbolic mental map: when that landscape was trespassed in a way that challenged the powers of the masculine state, or even the rural heteropatriarchal family, trespassers (most often women) were punished in severe ways.

At its most basic, the procreational geography of apartheid was one through which particular men (who were symbolically marked as heteromasculine) were granted limited mobility in urban spaces and women (symbolically marked a heterofeminine, or maternal) were immobilized in rural reserves. When women were found in apartheid's urban spaces, they either fulfilled domestic responsibilities (as maids, for instance) or ran the risk of strict social censure. Similarly, men who did not move through the geography of apartheid, opting rather to stay in the feminine rural reserves, sacrificed their heterosexual prowess. These men—young boys, old men, and the maimed—were clearly not "men enough" to move. Men who were able to hold kith and kin together, maintain masculine prowess, and by not moving to urban South Africa resist the geographical imperatives of apartheid, were deft, exceptional characters who performed a complex role that nevertheless drew on both heteropatriarchal "tradition" and modern apartheid-era heteropatriarchy:

> Janus-faced, the black patriarch is called upon to look inward—in on his family, to mobilise indigenous customs and practices for productive

purposes in accordance with African "tradition"—and to look outward to negotiate the demands of a changing economic dispensation in the "modern" idiom of his European landlord's alien culture. As Kas Maine once put it, successful negotiation of the economic and social intricacies of Triangle [north central South Africa] life demanded that he sometimes play at being "a chameleon amongst the Boers." (van Onselen 1996, 9)

Negotiating "African tradition" and apartheid's modernity (as well as their simultaneously complementary and contradictory visions of power in the black family) was the most important contract for men: if secured survival was possible. Unlike the celebrated Kas Maine, however, most men negotiated an implied heteropatriarchal covenant, between themselves and the state, by moving through apartheid's national space in rhythms dictated to by short-term labor contracts.

The Economic Implications of the Procreational Geography of Apartheid

Practically speaking and so as to achieve this apartheid geography, an estimated two million black women were sometimes violently, but always brutally, moved from their urban and rural homes throughout the country and relocated to the socially and economically marginal spaces known as reserves during apartheid (Platzky and Walker 1985). In those spaces, the work they performed was "domesticized" and devalued in terms of material reward. Given the extensive violence suffered by the black household generally and black women specifically, it is surprising that the resultant spatial "logic" and its straightforward gendered dimension has not received more attention. Unnoted is how apartheid's heteropatriarchal face demanded of relocated women an unpaid household labor and a range of informal occupations that guaranteed household survival. The meaning that work took (in terms of material reward) depended on its spatial relations. In other words, the devaluing of women's work was tied to a heteronormatized geography. Women's work, once relocated to the rural periphery, was marked as maternal, domestic household labor only and therefore unpaid. In essence, women were expected to re-create homes from a combination of their own unpaid activity and from the labor of recruited worker-husbands who traveled to and sent wages back from the urban heartland of South Africa. That women were then also expected to toil in a male-headed household, where the male household head was largely absent, requires that we suspend common sense. Is a maleless male-headed household still male headed? I think the answer is yes and no, but according to most literature on migration in southern Africa, the answer is always yes.

ha ha!

I believe that the complexity of the household is clearer outside heteronormative reasoning. Households were not male headed in a day-to-day sense. In fact most households were female headed in a real sense and increasing numbers are becoming so. Recent surveys tell us that South Africa's rural households are increasingly female headed (in both a de facto and a de jure sense) and those households are also increasingly likely to be impoverished (Klasen 2000). Should past and present trends lead us to conclude that that within the strictures of family life women were not subject to a wide-ranging set of patriarchal norms imposed by present older male relatives? No. But, these data should alert us to the possibility that women were active agents in their own lives and those of their children. The state's refusal to realize the complex history of these household relations later confounded its efforts to create sustainable infrastructure in rural reserves, later called homelands, Bantustans, and finally independent states.

Serial apartheid governments ignored the gendered complexity of African households that relied on male wages in the form of remittances, *as well as* the equally important free movement of women. However, the procreational economy of apartheid rendered symbolically maternalized women immobile. Very often, the actual support that emerged from male urban wages was not enough to support the male migrant worker, let alone give him "disposable" income he could send home to his family. As a result women were forced to find other means of household support. Both work-seeking and formally employed women usually committed spatial transgressions (if only temporarily) by rejecting the dictates heteropatriarchal apartheid laws designed to immobilize were "punished" in numerous ways for breaking these laws

One example shows how black women as sexual objects were constructed in the spaces they inhabited or moved through. A cursory glance at the well-documented Section 10 rights reveals how women were forbidden from moving through urban space unless they moved in accordance with the dictates of the procreational economy; unless black women were in search of or holding a domestic job that drew on their symbolic maternal sexuality, or in the company of men as either daughters or wives, they were unsanctioned. Black women, once employed in domestic service, soon discovered a battery of laws and policies intended to monitor their urban movements:

> All domestic workers have to be registered. Those who are migrants on one-year contracts may have their contracts renewed as long as they remain in the same job. As with other African migrants, changing jobs requires that the new employer makes a special application to a local administration board, proving that no African local labour is available. Thus the effect of this legislation is to impose an embargo on the entry of unskilled African women into "white" urban areas and to bind domestic workers to their present employers. Losing their job could well mean forced removal to the teeming rural slums of the homelands.
> (Cock 1989, 5)

Black women who did not involve themselves in maternal domestic work (either in their own rural homes, or in white urban homes) were constructed in terms of their sexuality in public: the black whore.

Recent reports to the Truth and Reconciliation Commission support this contention. Quoted in Antjie Krog's *Country of My Skull* (1998), Thenjiwe Mthintso, chairperson of the Gender Commission, opened a special hearing on abuses of women with the following:

> Behind every woman's encounter with the Security Branch and the police lurked the possibility of sexual abuse and rape. Some activists say they sometimes didn't know which was worse—the actual assault or dealing with the constant fear and isolated space of a cell. When they interrogated, they usually started reducing your role as an activist. They weighed you according to their own concepts of womanhood. And they said you are in custody because you are not the right kind of woman—

you are irresponsible, you are a whore, you are fat and ugly, or single and thirty and you are looking for a man.

And when whatever you stood for was reduced to prostitution, un-paid prostitution, the license for sexual abuse was created. Then things happened that could not happen to a man. Your sexuality was used to strip away your dignity. (1998, 178–79)

I quote at length from these findings because they reveal the life-threat-ening sanctions that women faced when they step outside the bounds of heteropatriarchy. While Mthintso's remarks underscore the risks she en-countered as an activist, at least the threat of sexual violence was experi-enced by mobile black women in most encounters with the state. The following account describes how women traveling under the conditions of apartheid faced two patriarchally entrenched threats of violence:

For my mother, travel was hazardous. If she traveled without men, she would be stopped by the police. This was always very dangerous for her. When she did travel with another man who was not directly related to her, she was also afraid to be alone with him on long, quiet parts of the road between here and Msinga. . . . She left us at home in 1955, 1961, 1968. For me, traveling is still hard but not so hard. Traveling by taxi or bus is now dangerous because of strangers, overcrowding, and speed. Hmph! The speed—it will kill us.[1]

The respondent sets her own experience apart from that of her mother's. Latter-day travel technologies, like taxis and highway infrastruc-tures between KwaZulu-Natal and the urban hinterspaces, have created another threat to women traveling in contemporary South Africa. Con-temporary dangers notwithstanding, the respondent's description of the threats of sexual violence negotiated by her mobile mother some thirty years ago might be read as evidence of how influx control laws helped to lay a restrictive heteronormative architecture in place. With time, that ar-chitecture would become the flimsy foundation of the apartheid system. As trespassers on the roadways of apartheid, women travelers ran risks that ranged from sexist intimidation to acts of sexual violence.

The uninterrogated effect of that legislation is an urgent challenge to urban policymakers and planners in contemporary South Africa, because mobility in South Africa has a raced and gendered legacy. The absence of a sustained intellectual examination of women's travel under the conditions of apartheid reveals how seldom women are imagined as mobile subjects. This omission is unfortunate as it blinds contemporary planners to possible avenues out of apartheid's landscape. A contemporary study in Ghana, for example, showed that one of the simplest means of alleviating rural poverty is through the provision of low-cost and safe transportation for rural women (Doran 1990).

As the lives of resistant mobile women come to bear on the history of apartheid, it is evident that support generated by women's "invisible" labor quite often resulted in a reversal of the supposed support that flowed from gainfully employed male relatives. By providing food, clothing, and sometimes financial support and emotional sustenance, millions of women reversed the pattern of dependence that apartheid architects publicly articulated (for recent examples of work on women and the migrant labor system, see Bozzoli 1991; Ramphele 1993; Miles 1993). These lives testify to the rejection of the state-sanctioned and normatized (which meant immobilized) heteropatriarchal standard.[2]

It is also important to realize that the degree to which women's lives were consciously regulated by the state in this way was neither constant nor transhistorical. During certain periods, women's formal employment (domestic or otherwise) was actively discouraged. During other phases the state's explicit policies are not as clear. Despite the ever changing relationship between black women and the state, black female sexuality and its relationship to labor was *always* used to support the migrant labor practice in general and the hostel system in particular. It is on this broader portrait of heterosexual rendering that the migrant worker hostel emerges.

The hostel system was a set of sociospatial relations, mutually constituted through heterosexual relationships, that dictated how and where work could be performed and to what end—that is, only men could live in it and move through its spaces. This does not suggest that women toiled at home in support of the apartheid regime. Rather, women relate to the hostel system in South Africa by way of a complex heteropatriarchal matrix that is shaped by power within the family, the state's manipulation of what it fantasized were heteropatriarchal familial relationships that sustained a racialized regime, and black South African women's responses negotiated within the rural household. To ignore this interplay of socio-spatial relations is to overlook one of the more significant processes within apartheid history and the contemporary state today. While the gendering of social space has been examined to some extent in South Africa (e.g., Friedman and Wilkes 1986; Robinson 1992), the spatiality of household survival strategies as a form of black women's resistance has not.

One dimension of that household struggle was black women's spatial transgression of apartheid laws by moving into hostel space. Interestingly, South Africa's apartheid managers absolutely and vehemently denied the physical presence of women in hostels until the early 1990s. By the time of this research, which was initiated in 1993 and completed in 1996, apartheid had collapsed. To admit to the presence of women in hostels at that late stage served only to reveal yet another place where apartheid had been unsuccessful. Despite the collapse of apartheid, however, the ways in which women living in hostels were reflected in the unquestioning sexist newspaper accounts served to underscore the way in which hostel spaces apparently reduced women to mere objects and, more specifically, sexual objects. What the following newspaper accounts reveal to us is the hidden (almost wink-wink, nudge-nudge) procreational geography of apartheid:

> The notorious KwaMadala Hostel in the Vaal has been implicated in yet another major scandal in which young girls have been held captive and abused as sex slaves by hordes of lusty inmates. (*City Press*, 2/16/92)

> Another Weekend of Fun and Romance in Sebokeng
>
> Stories have begun to emerge about women who are held captive inside hostels for two, three or four days. They are repeatedly raped by a variety of men, and beaten if they resist. They are then forced to clean and tidy up after all the debauchery they participated in. They are then required to cook for the men. (*Vrye Weekblad*, 4/8/92)

These newspaper accounts are shocking (or not) because they suggest that the raped and sexually harassed women somehow deserve their fate. There is no sympathy here for female spatial transgressors. The headline on the second piece conflates vile human rights abuses and "fun" and "romance" and in so doing attests to an unabashedly heteronormative worldview.

One way to examine the fate but also the responses of women to urban influx control is to locate their spatial movements on the procreational geography of apartheid. The occupation of hostel space on either a permanent or temporary basis always took place at great personal cost, but usually produced some economic benefit.

Clearly hostels are nonstatic spaces and their continual negotiation and reinvention by authorities and residents has always shaped their histories. For the sake of clarity I have loosely organized a history of women's mobility in South Africa into seven periods. These epochs, however, are defined by broader heteromasculine political and economic changes that took place in South Africa, not the feminized politics of daily life, which are as important. Note, however, that women's relations to the economy changed and that the actual time periods are of less importance than the process that occurred.

Inscribing Heterosexuality in Time and Space: Crafting the Procreational Geography of Apartheid

The South African feminist historian Julia Wells argues that "women's resistance to or compliance with influx control was generally shaped by household structures, divisions of labor and alternative forms of generating family income" (1993, 4). A women's history of influx control in South Africa, shows how the legal restrictions women encountered were quite different to the restrictions encountered by men. Throughout the 1960s, legal restrictions forced women to confront the contradictions of apartheid as they swept their kitchens on empty stomachs, cooked food of diminishing nutritional value, and took care of hungry children. While performing these unpaid household chores in far-flung rural reserves, it became evident to many of them that household economic survival *also* required their formal employment. What Wells and others leave unexplored is how the constructions of the black family and the roles of the black women within that institution came to be unquestioningly and unilaterally heterosexual.

Whether these sexed/gender dimensions were intended or not, the gendered effects of influx control were historically important to the implementation of these policies during all the phases of South African's economic development. Evidently for almost two hundred years, indigenous and black women in southern Africa experienced tightening and loosening strangleholds on their spatial movement and hence economic activity. The history of that mobility is also an account that underscores the *threat* that black maternally encoded female bodies posed at different points in time. The intimidating ability to produce children who could either support or challenge the myth of racial purity meant that black women in particular found themselves shunted through landscapes that would ensure a "racially pure" progeny.

Urbanization Policy, 1800–1920: Colonial Policy and the Transition from Farming to Mining

Influx control was intended to control the flow of migrant labor in South Africa. In varying guises influx control has been part of the South African condition for over two hundred years. Dating back to 1809, for example, the Caledon Code in the Cape Colony limited the free movement of Khoi and San servants. Throughout the 1800s, white farmers in the Western Cape region solved their periodic labor shortages with male and female contract workers from the present-day areas of Ciskei, Transkei, Namibia, and Mozambique (Wentzel 1993). During this time and well into the twentieth century a successful black peasant society coexisted with white commercial farming (Bundy 1972). An intended consequence of earlier influx control policies was to impoverish black peasants and transform them into waged labor. With the emergence of a capitalist economy in South Africa demanding cheap disposable labor on short-term contracts, the early foundations of a procreational economy began to emerge in South Africa. By requiring black South African men and women to mother and father, practically and symbolically, in particular legislated locales, the procreational economy began to produce some of the heterospatialities of the apartheid landscape. Early on, the resulting flows of people and constructions of places sought to regularize a temporally and spatially controlled form of heterosexual desire: men were to live temporarily in cities, women were to remain in the countryside while heteropatriarchal desire and responsibility strung across space and time secured and stabilized that economy.

The emergent mining economy of the late nineteenth and early twentieth centuries demanded cheap, unorganized, and easily disposable male labor. The discovery of diamonds at Kimberley in the 1860s, in particular, gave rise to an overnight demand for vast supplies of cheap, disposable labor. By temporarily locating men close to where labor was required but restraining black women from those sites of labor, an emergent procreational economy secured the cheap reproduction of labor. The heterosexual fantasy embedded in this particular policy was one that sought to "lure" men back to rural reserves once their contracts expired. Black women's sexed bodies became bait in this white-constructed, black heterosexual fantasy.

Black women, through their bodies, were constructed either as the loci of desire, fantasy, and paternal responsibility on a complicated procreational landscape or as the providers of maternal care and sustenance when sickness, injury, or old age resulted in male laborers' dismissals. Black women's spatially confined and heterosexually coded bodies became anchors on the apartheid landscape. These racial and sexed visions created a regional landscape that was easily replicated and expanded when a migrant labor system was eventually developed throughout the country and later, in collusion with local authorities, came to inform labor practices in the manufacturing sector sixty years later.

Patrick Harries (1990) has shown how the 1896 pass laws sharply curtailed freedom for blacks in the South African gold mines as well as the availability of housing for married miners. The erotic relationships that accordingly were established between adolescent boys and older migrant ethnic Shangaans from Mozambique serve to illustrate how sex and sexuality were shaped by migration policy. However, as Harries argues, this rearticulation of masculine erotic desire did not undermine indigenous patriarchal social structures in rural areas. Conversely, the spatial division of erotic desire (homosexual in urban mining centers and heterosexual in rural reserves) served to reproduce a vision of heterosexuality that shored up a particular black masculinity and femininity.

It should also be noted at this juncture that this analysis does not preclude many women from resisting these white and black male fantasies. For them these policies translated into a living economic nightmare. Indeed, Wells (1993) shows how women's resistance to their enforced immobility provided a hard-felt blow to South Africa's racialized economy in the 1950s. It should also be remembered that the strict enforcement of women's immobility occurred only in the mid-1960s.

mobility is resistence

By 1874 over ten thousand black male migrant mine workers were digging the diamond pits of Kimberley (Mabin 1986). The recruitment of this labor was not always voluntary, and very often male prisoners, guilty only of not possessing the correct influx control documentation, were used on the diamond fields. After securing a steady supply of labor, mining companies sought to ensure total control over the migrant laboring men who worked for them. Such draconian measures were seen as necessary to ensure that diamonds were not stolen and to curtail the high rate of desertion among workers, and so a compound or hostel system was set in place. The original plans emerged in a report on the control of mining labor in Brazil. In 1880 an official reported:

> The blacks are lodged in barracks, which are built in the form of a square, the outer wall being much higher than the inner-wall; the roof slopes inside. The entrance to the place is a by a large gate. . . . *Men* answer to their names while passing out at the gate in the morning and evening when entering . . . an overseer locks up the premises each night. . . . the Natives of South Africa, under European supervision are capable of being made almost—if not quite—as good as the Blacks of Brazil, provided they are dealt with in the same manner. (quoted in Mabin 1986, 12; emphasis mine)

The plan was soon implemented in Kimberley and later became the model upon which all migrant worker housing was developed. The spatial logic and gender specificity that informed the construction of these hostels created "spaces within which individuals were observed, partitioned, subject to timetables and disciplines, designed . . . as a form of moral architecture for the fabrication of virtue and hard work" (Crush 1992, 831). With the discovery of gold farther north, it was not long before a burgeoning Johannesburg also teemed with male migrant labor in need of control and accommodation. While hostels served to discipline and accommodate labor, these structures were also intended to operate as domestic spaces without women. Men undertook the litany of domestic chores in hostels, like food preparation and laundry. This transference of the demands of domesticity to the urban context without women created a series of contradictions for the emergent capitalist sector including a homoerotic system of patronage between older and younger men (Moodie 1994). However, even these acts of desire did little to disrupt the broader procreational economy. Indeed, as long as acts of same-sex desire took place within hostels only, the procreational economy of apartheid continued to operate without disruption. Following this thinking, we may also conclude that the procreational geography of apartheid was a landscape upon which same-sex desire was tolerated within certain times and spaces (see Elder 1998). In fact, patronage actually aided young men to accumulate the necessary bridewealth, as Dunbar Moodie has argued (for a critique of this position, see Achmat 1993).[3]

The all-male hostel system was set in place throughout the gold-bearing east and west axis of the southern Transvaal with Johannesburg at the center. Implicit in all this economic development was a subtext about male labor, women's labor, and a view about heterosexuality that would become regularized and ultimately normatized by the new divisions of space. The dismantling of the black household and its reassembly in terms that were surveyed and controlled reveals that, while the capitalist economy was emerging, so too were the early foundations of what was later the procreational economy of apartheid.

Prior to the 1890s women had not been subject to the pass laws. To that point, women's mobility had not been determined by work availability but rather by the availability of housing, income-generating alternatives, and family dynamics. With the discovery of gold, however, all that changed. The regulation of male labor and mobility was organized at the workplace and through the emerging hostel system. Although municipal regulations included both men and women, the laws were inconsistently applied. In areas where black domestic labor was scarce, some local authorities enforced regulations to ensure that black women sought domestic work. The precise way in which influx control was enforced, however, depended on the demand of the local domestic labor market. Ultimately, an overt interest in the control of women's mobility ceased. A rapidly expanding manufacturing sector focused attention on the demand for cheap male labor. As a result, from 1923 until 1956 black women were not technically required to carry passes and were not officially barred from urban areas (Wells 1993). A relatively successful (although over time declining) rural peasant economy guaranteed the reproduction of rural households. Accordingly, women were not forced to migrate in order to seek the means with which to maintain their households.

The everyday regulation of the black household during this period took place on a local scale. Arguably patriarchal in structure, the sexual politics of the household were not strung out over hundreds of miles, as would later be the case.

Urbanization Policy, 1920–1948: The Diversification of the Economy

Between 1920 and 1948 urbanization and influx control was constantly debated at a parliamentary level. The years between the two world wars witnessed a severe drought in rural areas, leading to the displacement of both black and white workers from the platteland (traditionally Afrikaner-owned farmlands in the Free State and the Transvaal) to the cities. In the first wave of rural-to-urban migration, displaced poor whites found un-skilled jobs in the commerce and industry that flourished during World War I. During the 1920s and 1930s, a similar growth in black urbaniza-tion resulted in more competition for jobs in cities. The shrinking num-ber of available jobs (brought about through the Depression of the early 1930s) and increasing numbers of black urban workers finally precipi-tated white job projectionist policies during the late 1930s.

During the 1920s and 1930s, no clear urbanization policy prevailed. Policy was at best piecemeal as it responded to both mining and indus-trial demands. What this lack of policy reveals is that no single economic sector had a decisive hold on government. First the Pact Government (1924) and then the Fusion Government (1929) under General Hertzog were born out of the need for political compromise. Throughout the 1920s and 1930s the concept of a national influx control was developed. Mining (replete with its well-organized hostel system) and agricultural interests argued for strong-arm interventionist state policies to remove all "surplus" Africans, including women and children, from the urban areas. Slowly, the contradictions of a localized heterosexual black family in urban areas emerged; steadily a spatially defined procreational economy emerged.

Only those workers who were absolutely necessary as wage laborers were to remain. Family members who were not gainfully employed in the formal labor market were relegated to the rural reserves, where it was assumed that the reproduction of the workforce would take place at a cheaper price. Evidence of this policy is clearly demonstrated from documented parliamentary debates and the resulting influx control amendments (South Africa 1934, 1936). Both the farming and mining sectors sought to benefit from such a policy in that it enabled both to pay extremely low wages to the workers.

After World War I and well into the late 1930s, Patrick Furlong (1994) argues, "white" Afrikaner Reformed Churches became increasingly exercised about interracial sex and marriage. This sexual panic (for examples of similar anxieties in North America, see Rubin 1984) contributed to the passionate fervor surrounding Daniel Malan's Purified National Party in the 1930s. These protracted moments of sexual anxiety and fantasy might be read as concern about the fragility of "racial purity." The close proximity and unchecked regulation of black and white bodies on the urban and rural landscapes of South Africa posed the risk of miscegenation. While it has been argued that the influx control policies and state interventions targeting blacks during this time sought to create preferential employment practices in favor of an impoverished Afrikaner proletariat (Harris 1987; Minnaar 1989), a documented and parallel "sex panic" muddies a simple race-based economic analysis. Rather, what appears is an emerging apartheid ideology that would come to craft a complicated economic landscape that also secured a racially pure and hence ideologically sound erotic, sexual body politic.

Low wages became a possibility for white capital because of the spatial fragmentation of the black heterosexualized family. In theory, immobilized and far-flung women and children were rendered dependent by way of the heteropatriarchal system of economic and social patronage. In reality, of course, women found that beyond contributing to the family through unpaid informal domestic labor, they were also under pressure to pursue remunerated employment in nonhome and sometimes urban places requiring them to trespass the heterosexualized geography of apartheid. With the growing demand for cheap masculine labor in the mining sector and a slowly crystallizing urbanization policy, the expressly gendered nature of influx control began to take shape. The cheap reproduction of black male labor in hostels became intertwined with the spatially separate, but nonetheless crucial, labor of female relatives who remained at home.

A growing industrial sector, however, showed a clear preference for leaving urbanization uncontrolled, subject to fluid labor market conditions. By paying higher wages than other sectors, industry was able to attract labor without coercion (Crush, Jeeves, and Yudelman 1991). Industry soon set about imitating the hostel system that mining capital had put in place to offset the labor reproduction costs of urban industries. While the intent was slightly different, industrial hostels too relied on and helped to deepen the heterospatializing apartheid landscape.

The establishment of an urban hostel system for manufacturing-employed workers was the result of joint efforts from local authorities and the manufacturing sector. Collaboration between local municipalities and the manufacturing sector, it was argued, was necessary to guarantee a reliable and steady flow of labor. Along with these local initiatives, a pattern of increasingly restrictive pass laws emerged from 1923 to 1937, which included some limited provision for the control of African women. This legislation, however, lacked enforcement mechanisms and accomplished little beyond the political appeasement of white voters. This non-enforcement suggests that the legislation was largely symbolic, calming white economic, sexual, and racial anxieties of the time. While the more panoptic mining compounds were regulated by mine contracts, male municipal hostel residents gained access to hostels only if they secured employment from any one of a number of employers in urban centers. Unlike the mining hostel system, which sought to create a steady and constant supply of labor, workers living in municipal hostels were more often at the mercy of the demands and profit cycles of the local labor market. Accordingly, the populations of municipal hostels during this time, while male, were less secure in their claim to urban shelter.

With South Africa's entry into World War II, industry boomed and in

b/c
Indust
booming
was

the early 1940s a free-flowing labor market nearly took over. Government, reflecting the preferences of the industrial sector, experimentally suspended pass laws (then applicable only to black men) in 1942. During the war a massive influx of blacks to the cities created pressure on limited nuclear family housing for black workers in urban areas. With the relaxed influx control policies in effect, yard communities emerged in the inner cities of South Africa. In some ways, the "yards" served to heighten white anxieties about "appropriate family housing" and were early precursors to the hostel communities that emerged in response to a relaxed influx control during the late 1980s. Although somewhat romanticized today, the yard communities of the 1930s (Hellmann 1935; Koch 1981) and places like Sophiatown, near Johannesburg (Hart and Pirie 1984), were also an attempt by women and men to negotiate survival by relocating to urban settings. In fact a close reading of Hellmann (1948) reveals that the residents of Rooiyard lived lives that flagrantly challenged ideas about ethnic and racial purity. Interracial marriages and nonheteronormative relations characterized many Rooiyard residents' lives. Ellen Hellmann admits to preselecting her "one hundred Bantu families," but even that effort requires qualification. Like dozens of scholars who would follow her dubious example (see discussion of Minnaar 1993, Sitas 1996, and Mamdani 1996 in chapter 6), Hellmann surgically shaped her sample to reflect a heteronormative ideal: "By 'family' I mean a complete household consisting of a husband, wife and, usually, children. Whether the man and woman forming this household had entered into some form of recognized marriage (recognized marriage includes religious marriage, civil marriage, and Native Customary Union) or whether their union was not legally sanctioned did not affect my choice. Widows, widowers, bachelors and unmarried women, whether childless or not are not included" (1948, 13). Clearly Hellmann's study is troubling because it chooses to erase the lives of individuals who do not fit her heterosexual model. However, it is Hellmann's particularity that also raised eyebrows in official circles. By selecting this particular group she inadvertently raised the very issue that urban policy architects feared most: interracial heterosexual mixing. It was not long before Rooiyard was destroyed. Urban racial integration, mostly among Coloured, Indian, and black urban citizens, was short lived. Harsh criticism from Afrikaner rural work-seeking migrants, who were also an emerging white political voting bloc, and from the mining sector, as well as a reported increase in crime in the cities resulted in the reintroduction of passes in 1945. The timing, of course, was also a function of a declining demand for black labor at the close of World War II.

The agricultural economy found itself in competition for labor with the booming industrial sector. The agricultural sector's dissatisfaction with the government's ability to ensure their labor supply is one explanation for the National Party's victory in the 1948 election. During and after the election, the National Party (NP) employed a racialized rhetoric that gave priority to the needs of Afrikaans-speaking white farmers, but also served the needs of an essentially English-speaking South African–owned industrial sector. The result was a Nationalist Party victory in 1948 and with it the legal entrenchment of apartheid:

> The NP came to power in 1948 on an "anti-capitalist" platform, whose proclaimed apartheid policy promised drastic state intervention in the functioning of labour and other markets. . . . to the surprise of many of its business opponents, even NP extremists like Native Affairs Minister Verwoerd proved remarkably amenable to the requirements of non-Afrikaner business. The overall effect of NP policies was exactly the opposite of that feared by the Chamber of Commerce. Under the governance of this "anti-capitalist" regime, the South African economy grew more quickly than any other capitalist economy except Japan during the 1950s and 1960s. (O'Meara 1996, 80–81)

While the era ended with a National Party victory there were also signs that unchecked economic growth in South Africa had created a permissive moral climate among recent white urbanites. The exhaustive detailing of the fraying of the white procreational economy is reflected in the research findings of Louis Freed. His published work *The Problem of European Prostitution in Johannesburg* (1949) documents, among other things, a rise in male homosexuality, prostitution, and masturbation in postwar white urban South Africa. It is no coincidence then that the National Party was able to come to power by drawing on the heteropatriarchal imagery of Afrikaner nationalism, fermented in the disenfranchised consciousness of the rural Afrikaner for most of the century (McClintock 1995) and inflamed by a "sex panic."

Policy, 1948–1985:
Fall of the Apartheid State

t Party regime brought with it an unprecedented level of the enforcement of a complex web of control measures r and black and white sexuality, something that had been lacking in the previous three decades. By 1952 legislation to implement stringent controls had been drafted (for detailed analysis of this period see Posel 1991). This included the extension of passes to women on a comprehensive national basis for the first time under the provision laid out in the Natives (Abolition and Co-ordination of Documents) Act of 1952 as well as the parallel development of the Sexual Immorality Act. The first of these pieces of legislation represented the key mechanism for channeling labor into the various sectors of the economy. The Native Laws Amendments Act of 1952 and amendments to the Urban Areas Act defined who was allowed (and who was not) to live and work in urban areas. Section 10 of the latter act stipulated the terms under which Africans would be considered permanent urban residents. The new legislation stated that a woman could never gain this status unless she or her husband could prove ten years of uninterrupted urban work. Added to this burden of proof was the stipulation that rural women could enter the urban areas to seek work for themselves only in the company of a male relative. Furthermore the job-search visit could not exceed forty-eight hours. Accordingly it is obvious that the pass system was put in place to discourage the flow of urbanward migrants, unless they fulfilled the able-bodied, masculine, and employed criteria laid down in the legislation. It is within this state-sponsored heteropatriarchal maze that novelist Elsa Joubert described Poppie Nongena's struggles:

> When she came to the office in Nyanga to change her pass, because her work extension had run out, My Strydom said: As the law stands now, I must give you a phumaphele. That's what the say in the location for: You must get the hell out, you must go away.
>
> The law was strict that the wives of men who had not been in the Cape fifteen years or hadn't worked ten years for the same boss must be sent back to their homes.

> But where to must we be sent back? Said mama. They brought us
> to Cape Town from Lamberts Bay. . . . Do you want to send me to
> Kaffirland? I belong to this land with these people here. I was born here
> and grew up here. (1985, 140)

The codification of women's immobility unless accompanied by a heterosexually defined relation (brother, father, son) set in place a strict system of moral and political surveillance. Passes that documented local authority permission to move, in conjunction with the hostel system, were used in a number of ways. First, the hostel system aided the new influx control measures by lowering the cost of reproducing male urban workers who had the right to work in urban areas. The "surplus" population (by which was meant the unemployed, women, children, the aged, the maimed, and the disabled) were shipped to "homelands," where they were superexploited in low-paying agricultural-sector jobs. By contrast, the urban mining and industrial sectors could selectively draw on a steady supply of cheap, masculine labor. To expedite that process, labor bureaus were established in the rural areas (for a poignant account of rural labor recruitment practices, see Pinnock 1981 and D. Gordon 1991). Classical critiques of apartheid have argued that the physical displacement of the unemployed, women, children, and the elderly to the rural areas constituted the creation of a reserve army of labor that kept urban wages low (Bundy 1972).

While the reserve army of labor argument explains part of the process, the well-rehearsed and now classical critique fails to show how women's formal and informal work supplemented the low urban wages that men received. This critique fails to acknowledge the broader outlines of the procreational economy that were being drawn at the time. The traditional account ties women to rural reserves, posits their labor as only informal and domestic, and thereby operates within Butler's previously discussed heterosexual matrix of intelligibility.

The new influx control measures were intended to restore levels of profitability in the declining agricultural sector. Drought and a depopulation of white, small-scale farms proved to be a crisis for the agricultural sector throughout South Africa. To reverse this process and shore up declining agrarian profitability, the state's gendered policy offered cheap and physically restricted female laborers to white farmers as a possible way out of the rural crisis. While this strategy did draw working black rural women into the formal rural waged economy, policies of spatial fixity that targeted black women specifically secured the rurality of black families. Indeed, for white nation builders challenged by declining white agrarian profitability and anxious at the threats of interracial heterosex, fantasies about heterosexual desire between sexually marked black bodies, and planner's faith in the strength of that attraction across space and time, secured in their own mind the feasibility of family-fragmenting influx control. It is only by way of this "logic" that the contradictions of apartheid can be reconciled: destroy but retain the black family.

The state sought to redefine the role of rural black men and the terms of rural patriarchy so as to serve the demands of racial capital. The altering of his position, therefore, can be seen as an effort to engineer gender relations in particular ways.

For African women, the prospect of these controls was highly threatening. The implementation of influx control came at a time when new employment possibilities were opening up for women in urban areas. The number of women in industrial employment had grown under the wartime conditions of the early 1940s and continued throughout the 1950s. These jobs in the formal sector paid much more than did domestic service or farm labor, which had been the traditional employment sectors for black women. For many women, passes also meant restrictions on their movement into and out of formal- and informal-sector employment in conjunction with the changing needs of their families. The options they had enjoyed because of their freedom of movement over the years were lost.

A history of women's resistance to influx control reveals how women had to combine income-generating activities with household responsibilities (Wells 1993). Before influx control measures, black households had relied on the free movement of women between rural subsistence and urban labor (formal or informal). By forcing women into rural subsistence or the low-paying agricultural labor market, influx control severely reduced women's income-generating abilities. Simply put, the new policy restricted the movement of women by linking legal urban status to formal urban employment; the policy thereby became the immediate site of a struggle for survival.

Before the 1960s, the negotiation of household survival for women had been premised upon women's free movement between urban and rural areas, formal and informal economic sectors, and farming and industrial labor markets. Under the new influx control policy, men found themselves pressured into wage labor by a collapsing and overpopulated rural peasant economy. In the transition to wage labor, male family members exchanged a single form of production, namely agricultural work, for another, namely industrial labor. Women, in contrast, experienced conflicts between their traditional heteropatriarchal responsibilities (child rearing, cooking, cleaning, and farming) and the economic responsibilities demanded by the patriarchal apartheid state. Black women's daily lives revolved around defining a balance between domestic duties and income-generating activities in either the formal or informal economy. Under the new influx control regulations, women's ability to float between nonhome places and job markets was challenged. Within this context demonstrations by black women against the pass laws are understandable (Wells 1993). While Cherryl Walker (1991) has argued that women's resistance to influx control was undertaken to defend female domesticity, I am suggesting instead that resistance marks how women insisted on having a say over the terms of their relations to the wage labor market.

As time wore on, the central apartheid state began to divest itself of influx control regulation and enforcement. Once again local authorities found themselves having to apply state policy. With the establishment of local administration boards in 1973, the lands on which black towns were built in urban areas were transferred to the boards for control. At the same time hostels in the township also became the property of the local boards.

Urbanization Policy, 1985–1994: The Collapse of the Apartheid State

During the late 1980s attempts by yet another apartheid state to stem the flow of urban-bound migrants proved futile. In an attempt to regain control of the mounting number of illegal urban residents, the government embarked on a so-called orderly urbanization policy (Hindson 1987; Robertson and McCarthy 1988). One of the most bizarre examples of "apartheid geography" that developed during that time involved the establishment of black local authorities. These established bodies, the Administration Boards, administered some urban land in townships and thereby absolved the central state of its direct responsibility to house black urban dwellers. Because hostels often fell outside the jurisdiction of these newly established black local authorities, hostels became the responsibility, by default, of white-run regional Administration Boards, who in turn gave the money generated from hostels to local black authorities to upgrade and manage black towns. Slowly the conditions in hostels began to decline as the money they generated was funneled into township upgrading. In some instances the health of hostel dwellers was jeopardized (Ramphele 1993). The crisis reverberated throughout the region. People began to challenge the strictures of apartheid's geographies in other ways too. At the same time, for example, and as a direct consequence of the housing shortage created by the wave of urbanization, residential segregation in high-density apartment neighborhoods also began to break down (Elder 1990).

As part of the apartheid state's restructuring in the face of an increasing crisis, influx control was scrapped because, among other reasons, the cost of enforcement proved exorbitant. Instead, the government embarked on establishing a number of growth poles around the country in an attempt to redirect urbanward migration. Growth poles, also called border industries, became the focus of the apartheid government's attempt to stem the tide of black urbanization. Further, these low-wage maquiladoras —like factories on the veld—aimed to attract foreign investors, many of whom were withdrawing from the South African economy because of political uncertainty and an ANC-inspired United Nations-led trade embargo against the apartheid state. The South African government poured millions of South African rands into establishing industrial parks near many of the borders of the "independent states." Despite these attempts, little changed and the numbers of people migrating to cities simply increased. With the increasing deregulation of hostel space, increasing numbers of vagrants began to settle in hostels (*Daily Dispatch,* 6/2/92).

Women's organized resistance to influx control measures has a long history (Walker 1991; Wells 1993). The movement of women into hostel spaces must be understood in the context of the importance women attached to free movement and the extent to which these controls were violated by women. The occupation of hostels by women since the mid-1980s, when influx control measures were relaxed, is a clearly recognizable moment, because of its public nature, in the history of linkages between women, hostels, and evolving influx-control policies. Of equal importance is an appreciation of the spatiality of hostels and influx control. An apartheid history created a racialized and gendered sense of place. It is important, then, to examine the movement of women into hostels as a spatial act. What follows is a partial examination of how places and meanings were gendered, as part of apartheid's spatial engineering.

The Gendering of Influx Control and Hostels: A Sociospatial Perspective

The articulation of influx control took place on at least three levels. The national, local, and household levels intersect in several ways. I have elected to examine the sociospatial relations at the household level because of the significant roles that women perform on this scale. It is also on this scale that changes in the regulation of intimate daily life are writ most large and their connection to national policy most clear. It is, after all, at the household level that the geographical "elasticity" of the household is most obvious. On the household scale we find that women in particular negotiated preexisting and imposed heteropatriarchal systems to bring about family survival. Most often the negotiating of those sometimes complementary and contradictory social systems took place through space and most often by moving.

An examination of household strategy reveals a detailed interplay of national and local policy, while providing a level of agency to those (in this case women) within the household who negotiate ways around these policies on a daily basis. Given the spatial nature of the argument that follows, it remains important to examine exactly how the three scales interlocked and reinforced both the racialized capitalist economy and the racialist procreational economy.

The Gendering of Rural Domestic Space

To assume that the underrepresentation of women in the urban area between 1948 and 1985 reflects their nonparticipation in the institution of migrant labor is incorrect. Relegated to the rural reserves, many women acted out their lives in rural households. This spatial division of labor, remember, served to reinforce the procreational underpinning that fueled the economy. Very often these mothers, sisters, and wives struggled—successfully and sometimes unsuccessfully—to support and reproduce impoverished families. Women's work (assigned by way of maternal responsibility, located in rural areas and thereby devalued in monetary terms) in fact supported male relatives in urban areas, very often reversing the theoretical pattern of dependence (Moodie 1994). At home they struggled to keep families intact, providing moral and physical sustenance for children and sick or aging relatives, or those men that could not fulfill the procreational or labor mission (e.g., older men, maimed men, young boys). These private spaces, however, also provided women with the tools with which to empower themselves and to confront apartheid in other ways. In the context of the United States, but expressing a tension similar to the one described above, bell hooks argues, "Since sexism delegates to females the task of creating and sustaining a home environment, it has been primarily the responsibility of black women to construct domestic households as spaces of care and nurturance in the face of the brutal harsh reality of racist oppression, of sexist domination" (1991, 44). Also, by locating women in a heteropatriarchal configured household, acts of survival or strategies of resistance (sometimes the same thing) can also be interpreted as acts against the prevailing heteropatriarchal household structure and the state. In South Africa the male migrant worker's experience is etched onto the urban landscape and reflected in official documents. Public and visibly masculine hostels and sprawling industrial areas were the life worlds of millions of male migrant workers. Unlike the lives of male migrant workers, women's lives in rural areas remain undocumented and therefore hidden. South African researchers with the aid of gendered analyses began to hear women's accounts. *Women of Phokeng* by Bozzoli shows how women actively participated in the migrant labor system in South Africa. This text weaves a tapestry of South African women migrant's lives:

Who could have looked after my children whilst I was working in Johannesburg? Tell me, who would have been prepared to carry one's load, carrying one's children piggyback style whilst one was away on employment? . . . Am I a fool to abandon my children whilst I am still living. A person who neglects her children and deserts them for employment is an idiot. What does she think about them? I find such people's actions to be mind intoxicating. What does such a person think about her own flesh and blood which she has given birth? (quoted in Bozzoli 1991, 122)

The quote shows how apartheid policy shaped not only the labor force, but also male and female heterosexual subjectivities. Clearly, female responsibility is located within assumptions about motherhood and the attendant procreational expectations that underpinned apartheid. South Africa was suffused with highly gendered assumptions concerning the roles of individuals within the heteropatriarchal family structure. Further, for women, direct participation in migrant labor was not a prerequisite for involvement in the migrant labor system. What remains unexamined are the interconnected spatial relations of men's and women's relations to migration. Migration, household survival, and even future family housing design are all inherently spatial practices, and so a systematic analysis of these relations will benefit from a spatial focus and in some ways underscore the interconnected way in which they come together.

The Gender Struggle over Hostel Space

The sexual gendering of the apartheid landscape provides a number of spatial scenarios for us to examine. The masculinization (an attendant sexualization) of hostel space is one example of how apartheid, gender, sex, and space come together. Women living in hostels today provide evidence of the renegotiations and struggle over hostel space and its sex/gender meaning.

Within this apartheid structure, women have recently confronted and thus redefined and restructured the current experience of hostel life. Mamphele Ramphele (1993) provides a contemporary account of hostel life that includes both men and women as hostel residents. She demonstrates how micro and macro private and public spaces and the masculine and feminine meanings associated with those spaces make up the migrant work experience. Here I will extend that analysis by showing how women have always been part of hostel life, not only as residents but also as spatially removed domestic laborers under apartheid, and that their physical occupation of hostels today is a testament to that past. Furthermore, I hope to show that while Ramphele correctly identified the gendered nature of hostel life, her failure to relate those findings to sexuality has left the experiences of women's and men's interconnected lives somewhat untheorized. I would argue that there is a compelling reason to do so during the broader politics of transformation currently underway in contemporary South Africa.

As increasing numbers of women move into hostels across South Africa and some are evicted, the role and meaning of the hostel within the family has shifted. Particularly since increasing numbers of women have moved into hostels since the mid-1980s, the institutional assumption that hostels were exclusively masculine and public in nature has been shown to be unfounded. Despite these pioneering moves by women to renegotiate the gendered and sexed meanings of space in South Africa, their contributions to contemporary policy debates has been largely ignored.

Women's hidden histories of migrant labor and current experiences in hostels have significant impacts on current developments in South Africa. The exponential growth in the number of women who have migrated from rural areas to cities and into hostels since 1985 is simply one chapter that documents how women have negotiated influx control policies to retain household cohesion. An established literature has begun to document, albeit in a limited way, the role of migrant women in urban formal and informal settlements (e.g., see Goodlad 1996; Pikholz 1997; Mackay 1999). Hostels, on the other hand, present a unique South African challenge to prevailing thought on women and urban housing.

As part of the sex-gender history of migration and hostel life, the current violence is also important, not least because of how that violent history has systematically sidelined women's claims to housing in contemporary South Africa. Of note is the particularly masculinized way in which the violence has been portrayed in the media. The severity of the "hostel violence" was illustrated by two state-sponsored reports (South

Africa 1991; Minnaar 1993), both of which present the hostels as cellular, foreboding spaces in which the national politics of ethnic solidarity were forged. Seldom, if ever, has the hostel been discussed as an interconnected domestic space. Hostels can also be seen as domestic spaces within which the struggles of daily life are negotiated by men and women (in public or in private, sometimes in violent ways). Those domestic struggles around hostel spaces are at the center of an interconnected, albeit geographically far-flung, struggle for household survival.

Conclusion

In all areas of life, the effects of apartheid on women were significantly different from its impacts on men. In the early 1960s the struggle against apartheid was defined by women demanding the right to move freely within and around the cities of South Africa (Wells 1993). After influx control was finally abolished in 1985, the free flow of women to the cities created new challenges for women in urban settings, as the competition for housing and shelter became acute. What has remained undocumented is how these moments of resistance and changing migration patterns are negotiated at the level of the household.

Most black women soon discovered that their socially marginal position under apartheid frustrated their efforts to house themselves and their families. In contemporary South Africa the effects of the past are still felt and will be for some time to come. A history of discrimination against women in urban areas ensures that apartheid's procreational legacy remain in full force. It is therefore no coincidence that while women struggled for housing in the already overcrowded formal and informal housing markets, the internal demographics of the previously "all-male" hostels in South African cities changed too. Although hostels were built upon a sexed and thereby gendered assumption about the division of labor, the actual physical presence of women living in urban hostels is a relatively recent, albeit rapidly expanding, phenomenon.

To overstate the point and argue that the migrant labor system as practiced in South Africa resulted in a total exclusion of women from urban areas, and a total absence of men from rural areas, is incorrect. Many women did in fact move to the urban areas. An important consideration, however, is that women's experiences in either rural or urban areas were regulated by their roles and identities as black women under apartheid and their accordant relegation to the domestic sphere. Husbands, brothers, and sons, however, tended to play out their "apartheid identities" as migrant workers in the public space of the hostel, the factory, or the mine. The lives described above are the complicated roles performed by those that performed the ballet of daily life on apartheid's procreational landscape.

As argued above, migrant labor emerged out of a system that was at once contradictory, overlapping, and overdetermined in its vision of the black heteropatriarchal family. Both the colonial and apartheid state believed and promulgated the notion that men and women work to survive, but with one glaring exception: men get paid, women don't. A set of spatially engineered laws (influx control) created a cheap labor force that boosted the South African economy. The glue that held this system in place were the bonds of affection and desire between black men and women, sometimes real and sometimes informed by white fantasies and myth making.

As the history of apartheid is told, it is increasingly important to realize that it operated as a racist *and sexist* body of laws. Men and women's experiences of apartheid differed significantly. In order to realize these differences, it is important to examine assumed meanings connected to all spaces under apartheid. In the new South Africa defined by an unpacking of apartheid, it is therefore increasingly important to restructure society in all spheres. In keeping with all decolonization processes this involves remaking the spatial assumptions that underlie the social structure.

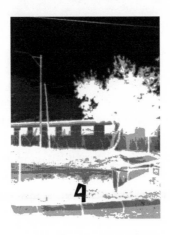

4

FORTRESSES OF FEAR

APARTHEID WAS premised upon a procreative tension: the spatial fracturing of the black family unit, but not its destruction. Designers of apartheid policy realized that by stringing black heteropatriarchal bonds of desire and responsibility across space and time, white wealth and the impoverished reproduction of black labor would be assured and secured. The intention was to restructure existing social relations and reconstruct a particular kind of familial heterosexuality across space and time. An example of the explicit attempt to socially engineer heteropatriarchy toward some profitable racialized end follows. Focusing on the Pedi, Sotho, Bhaca, Mpondo, Zulu, and Swazi, the commentator attempts to produce an intellectual justification for reengineering the sociology and geography of rural Africans: "For the uneducated tribesman, the greatest scope for altering his situation is by altering his position in the webs of social relationships in the tribal area" (Sansom 1974, 159). By reconfiguring heterosexuality across space, so the fantasy goes, heterosexual desire (between men and women), or heteropatriarchal bonds of affection (between mothers and sons, fathers and daughters, etc.) would guarantee the reproduction of the system. This spatial reconstruction of heterosexual relations took place by shaping individual family members' identities in "apartheid places" like the township, the homeland, or the migrant worker hostel. Influx control laws aimed to siphon husbands, fathers, brothers, sons, and uncles off into the urban industrial centers and to relegate wives, mothers, sisters, daughters, and aunts to the peripheral rural areas of South Africa. By fracturing families but not completely destroying them in that way, the apartheid state reconstructed black families' identities into functional heteropatriarchal identities and thereby functional worker identities—male wage workers and female unpaid laborers. Individuals who resisted or trespassed this neat heterospatialized geography, arguably, resisted apartheid; men who stayed on in rural areas or women who decided to move to urban areas without masculine permission challenged the sexual assumptions of apartheid or the procreational economy of apartheid. Taking her cue from the spatial script, one interviewee explained it thus: "The urban areas is not a place for women. We are always in danger here; there is no place built for us here. We should not be here. We have no right to say we want this, we want that."[1]

The changing character of hostels provides one spatial context for examining how the procreational geography of apartheid operated and continues to operate. Hostels are also sites where the procreational geography of apartheid was resisted. As the ultimate expression of an apartheid spatial form, hostels were also officially designated as heteromasculine spaces (although in actual fact this designation was somewhat ambiguous, as will be discussed below). While hostels were one site where apartheid identities were forged, hostels were, and continue to be, sites where family members (including women and children) resisted and co-opted the imposition of new identities that would have otherwise destroyed their household and family structures.

The "hostel family household" then is a process by way of a web of meanings for all South Africans that extends well beyond the barbed-wire fence of the hostel (see fig. 4.1). For all contemporary hostel dwellers (men and women), these meanings emerge as resultant vectors in a geometry of survival and resistance strategies, apartheid, and familial heteropatriarchal relationships. In what follows, we will see that the "official" intent of hostels—as an arsenal of disposable wage labor created by way of a familial rearticulation across space—was never passively accepted, or suc-

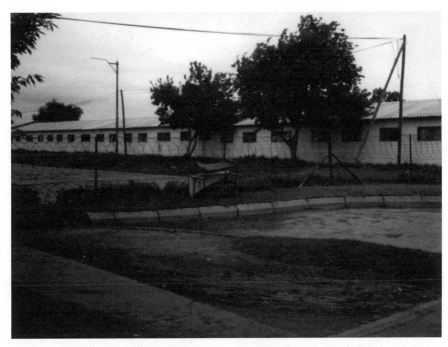

Fig. 4.1. Between 1990 and 1996 the hostel was separated from the township with a barbed-wire fence.

cessful in its mission. Instead, we see the municipal hostel, as an apartheid state–engineered ideal, was never realized because it was resisted, "invisibly" co-opted, and incorporated into an extended household structure by hostel dwellers.

The hostel did cut deeply into the South African psyche, changing black family life as it was known. However, the black family was not always shattered. That oversimplified break-up of the household suggested in much of the literature on hostels did not take place (e.g., Minnaar 1993). The terms of that struggle took place around the meaning of heterosexual familial relations in space; at times these heteropatriarchal assumptions were in line with those of the state; at other times women in particular resisted their imposition—resistance strategies of hostel dwellers, and women especially, that can be understood only once we accept that their response took shape around the struggle over sexed gender identity and survival at the household level. Although the contestation for meaning and identity between hostel dwellers and the state took place throughout the apartheid years, it was only in the mid- to late 1980s that the sexed and gendered nature of that struggle emerged visibly—in newspaper accounts and in the form of women occupying hostels.

As part of the effort to massage the apartheid landscape into a less oppressive spatial form, hostel conversion schemes have sparked an architectural controversy about the shape of future "family" housing in South Africa. However, in all these discussions, a heterosexual matrix has confounded all contemporary discussions of family as "heterosexual families": "Happiness is a home with his family" quipped a newspaper headline referring to a hostel migrant's future (*Star,* 3/10/93).

Proposals seldom acknowledge that families were always part of the hostel in a spatially fragmented way. Missing from proposals too was any recognition of female-headed "families" who had already moved into the hostels, preempting the official call. As a consequence, for women living in hostels postapartheid planning looked remarkably similar to apartheid planning. Their informal work lives, which balanced income and household responsibility, were still devalued, and their links to hostels, regardless of how they were upgraded, were still dependent on male relatives.

By the close of 1990 the then recently unbanned African National Congress, the South African Communist Party, and the South African government established an alliance that set R4 billion ($1.2 billion at the time) aside for these conversions. To manage the funds an independent trust was established (*Sunday Tribune,* 10/16/90; *Star,* 10/17/90). Proposals soon followed: "For each family unit in the hostel, one has to move 15 people. . . . To create facilities for the community, we recommended that the opportunity for small business be encouraged and that older disused buildings be used as workshops to generate self-employment. Hostel dwellers that were unemployed could be used as builders in modifying the hostels" (*Daily News,* 10/18/90). The findings of an unabashedly sexist architectural survey argued, among other things, that

> Three types of hostel dwellers were identified: The migrant worker who had invested in the homelands over a period of time and was not looking to settle in the city. Those with urban aspirations who could not afford to live in the township although they aspired to move and integrate with the community. Those men too insecure in their employment to

think about integrating into the community argued that they planned to return home. (*Daily News*, 10/18/90)

At best what these plans and proposals reveal is an effort to release some of the heterosexual tensions of desire across space and time: plans that permit women to stay overnight in hostels. It does not recognize the lived reality of female-headed hostel family households, hostel family households led by older men who are not husbands, or any household that does not present a procreational unit. This is astounding, given that these nonheteronormative and certainly less heteropatriarchally controlled family units presently live in many old hostels throughout South Africa. In fact, current debate around hostel conversions into family housing has reinforced the procreational geography of apartheid. In other words, it is only families who measure up to some apartheid-inspired notion of procreational worth who access housing today in old hostel spaces. Widows who head families, grandfathers who adopt AIDS orphans, and young unmarried parents of both sexes will not find adequate and affordable housing in contemporary South Africa. The tokoloshe, it would seem, is alive and well.

The linkages between areas of origin and the hostel are also at the core of the struggle for identity that hostel dwellers have experienced since the collapse of apartheid. The physical incarceration of hostel dwellers behind barbed-wire fences, and their symbolic imprisonment secured by a discourse that labels their living space as "Fortresses of Fear" (*City Press*, 6/30/91), "slaughter houses" (*City Press*, 6/21/92), and "primordial palaces of darkness" (*Citizen*, 4/30/92) isolated their urban experience. In the late 1980s and 1990s struggles over the meaning of hostels have marginalized hostel dwellers (by which I mean women and children as well as men) in such a way that the path is left open to a South African variation on postcolonial exploitation and ultimate genocide. Tragically, desperate living conditions, unsurpassed poverty even in South African terms, and the violent and politically motivated death of almost ten thousand persons in hostel-related violence since the mid-1980s support this claim. These debates reveal that for many South Africans during apartheid, the hostel was terra incognita; so in contemporary South Africa these spaces remain vulnerable to speculation, generalization, and stereotyping.

The urgent need to clarify issues surrounding the meaning of hostels has elicited numerous understandings and conceptualizations on the part of academics, government policymakers, and the disparate hostel dweller population itself. One of the first comprehensive studies of hostels by the postapartheid government (Minnaar 1993), in a collection tellingly titled *Communities in Isolation,* used an expensive and intricate sampling procedure of the "hostel population," but failed to draw any surprising conclusions. In part, the study was unsuccessful because it used generalized categories and variables that were informed by the apartheid past. For example, a person in the category *hostel dweller* was assumed to be male, black, and legally registered as a hostel tenant—an experience or identity that defines only a small percentage of hostel dwellers today.

We need to explore the ways in which a sexed and gendered analysis of spatial relations might succeed in overcoming the apartheid-inspired generalizations about hostels that plague current reform proposals. Once we examine the hostel from a sexed and gendered perspective, the hostel offers an important view of the contemporary black family. A sexed and gendered analysis uncovers hostels as sites of household resistance by drawing links to processes outside its physical structure. The hostel is not, and never was, simply the machinery of masculine exploitation. The hostel was, and still is, incorporated into the rural family structure.

To facilitate this theoretical examination of hostels as part of black households, I take the mutually constituted construction of identity and space as an entry point. Although identity formation is a highly complex web of relational categories that include ethnicity, age, physical ability, class, and so on, I focus on the racial, sexual, and gendered aspects of identity and space. When hostels are viewed through this lens, the increasing visibility of women in hostel space during the 1980s emerges as a flash point in the sexed and gendered history of hostel households.

We cannot take conceptions of race, gender, sexuality, and space for granted. The terms in and of themselves have produced an incredibly rich and complex set of arguments. What follows is a discussion of the debates that inform the theoretical underpinnings of this kind of research. Accepting the need to theorize the nature of hostel life, we can isolate the following set of questions as an organizing framework. First, why is the intersection of space and identity an appropriate departure point for theorizing the hostel? Second, which notions of space, and what aspects of identity are useful for informing an analysis of the hostel?

The Intersection of Space and Identity
as a Departure Point for Retheorizing Hostels

The history of apartheid is a history of spatial engineering (Cohen 1986). The forced removal of the black population from one place to another, the seizure and renaming of their land by the state, and the creation of "homelands" in deserted regions of the country are just some of the ways in which geography, and the meaning of place, informed the apartheid principle.

As a place, the South African hostel was charged with a sense-filled meaning for residents and a regulatory purpose for authorities. Unlike many other places under apartheid, however, that meaning and purpose revealed a "raced" and gendered face of apartheid that was less obvious in other settings. Within the spatial confines of the hostel walls, the state and capital collectively produced an idealized, cheap masculinized black male labor force. At the same time, the state barred women from the hostel's physical landscape, although as we will see, the ban did not exclude them from the hostel process. Instead the collusion between apartheid state policy and an emerging capitalist order relegated women in their roles as wives, daughters, mothers, and female laborers to the rural areas of South Africa.

In order to capture the way in which women's lives intersected with the hostel system in particular, we need to develop a sensitivity to place without "rigidifying" the analysis. Said argues that static ideas concerning space and the interlinkages between spaces has led to a "static notion of identity that has served to oppress and silence colonial and post-colonial subjects" (1993, xxv). Conditions under apartheid created static racial identities and then separated the population into static racialized spaces. By cracking the hard shell that encases personal and spatial identity in South Africa, we can identify shifting processes that relate to place and identity formation.

Terms like *race, sex,* and *space* need reexamining and careful deconstruction in a contemporary South Africa. For this reason I will employ a consciously antifoundationalist ontology. In other words what follows is a conceptualization of knowledge characterized by the recognition of the importance of the perspective of the knower (Guba 1990). In so doing, we are able to posit the fluidity of space and identity. Using that as a cornerstone to the argument, we will cut across and through many of the rigid identities like black and white, male and female, as well as "concrete" spaces (like hostels) that continue to express the postapartheid moment. By resisting the legacy of apartheid in this way, we will establish a framework for understanding the ways in which individual actors negotiate the identity-laden hostel terrain, by either yielding or challenging its constraints and opportunities.

Which Notion of Space Can Inform the Hostel Narrative?

Our examination of hostel spaces is grounded in Massey's notion (1993) of place as a process. The traditional static spatial conceptualization of the hostel fails to appreciate its interconnectedness to other places and processes that lie outside its immediate environs. The interrelationships between the hostel and other nearby or faraway spaces must inform a retheorization of the hostel. Running parallel and connected to the physical interlinkages are a series of nonphysical, or imagined, geographies that are of equal importance. The attraction of Massey's concept generally lies in her fluid sense of space, which draws on both the physical and imagined geographies of place. To achieve this purpose, she sketches a fourfold development of place.

First, Massey argues that conceiving of place as a process dispels its static character. Rather, places become constituted by the coalescence of social interactions (themselves processes) at specific locales. Through a vision of the hostel as a site of converging social relations, we transcend the narrow, state-imposed idea of the hostel as a purely physical building. Instead, processes like gender formation become intimately tied to its "placefullness."

The second point Massey makes concerns the fluid sense of space that informs her definition. She argues that places do not have divisions in the sense of divisions that frame simple physical enclosures. In particular, the appeal lies in the hostel as an unbounded physical space. Further, it allows us to examine the hostel as part of a series of other spatial relationships and linkages, like the spatially displaced rural household and family members. Thus the hostel becomes a process and not simply a place.

Third, Massey argues that places do not have single, unique identities;

rather, they are full of internal differences and conflicts. By examining the hostel place as a site of conflict, we can examine how these interpretations over meaning, future, occupancy, and history shape the hostel as a place.

Finally, Massey argues that by viewing place as a process, constituted by a network of meanings and relationships, we see how the specificity of place is continually reproduced. Accordingly, the hostel becomes a place that is related to other places through a network of interrelationships. Rather than isolating the hostel as a stark, physical reminder of apartheid, we can integrate the gendered realities of hostel life historically, into the larger apartheid plan and into the current redevelopment program that is underway in South Africa. Here, the hostel becomes a distinct mixture of national and local, historical and contemporary social relations. The juxtaposition of these relations specifically will result in the formation of place and the unique spatial identity that it represents.

Other South African geographers who study state-run hostels or private-sector regulated migrant worker compounds have also drawn on the sense of place that Massey proposes. Crush has remarked that "Massey's notion of power geometry has important implications for an empowering narrative of the compound" (1994, 314). He argues that in using Massey's concept of place we can in fact see how the hostel or compound is intimately tied to other spaces.

> It is these connections, as much as what went on directly within those spaces, that formed and transformed their character. This is clearly illustrated in the case of migrant workers. During the course of an average working year, *male migrants* inhabited a succession of subaltern spaces —rural homesteads, segregated trains, compounds, townships, slumyards, prisons. Their presence or absence significantly shaped the nature of those spaces. Their own consciousness and culture was made by their highly mobile existence and experience of a succession of places. (314; emphasis mine)

Where Crush (1994) uses the metaphor to examine those who were legally recognized and visible (i.e., male workers), here we can extend its usage to include those who were not present but nevertheless connected. It is at this point that a gendered analysis of the hostel dynamic informs our understanding. With the aid of Massey's power geometry, we can transcend the narrow state-imposed historical definition and meaning of the hostel and investigate how women and men in relation to each other and family structure contributed to the hostel system.

Other African gender scholars have used the analytical insights of the interconnectedness of space in revealing ways. Mamphele Ramphele, in an address entitled "Empowerment and the Politics of Space" (1989b), calls for a focus on the spatial relations of daily life as a possible avenue for gendered South African socioeconomic understanding. Ramphele's own work (1986, 1989a, 1993) among hostel residents of the Western Cape demonstrates the incisive strength of a spatially sensitive gendered argument: "The common denominator of space allocation in the hostels is a bed. . . . it is the basis for relationships within the hostels, between different hostels, and between hostels and places of employment. One's very identity and legal existence depend on one's attachment to a bed" (1993, 20). While she emphasizes the constraints exerted on hostel dwellers by the limited spaces they inhabit, she also argues that within these constraints people have managed to find room to maneuver and resist apartheid.

The shifting social relations over space (in this case outside of South Africa) are also revealed in Schmidt 1991, where the colliding forces of patriarchy, race, and class emerge differently in different places throughout colonial Rhodesia. Luise White (1990) has demonstrated how urban women in colonial Kenya renegotiate gender relations through access to housing by examining the importance of the social context that was Nairobi. Although not making an explicitly spatial argument, she provides yet another example of an explicitly gendered and implicitly sociospatial set of relations on a micro scale.

Microspatial relations are particularly intriguing in the current migration process in South Africa because the spatiality of everyday life and changing relations are most obvious at this level. Ramphele (1989a) demonstrates the linkages between places, showing how certain areas within the hostels have historically been proclaimed as male space, echoing the patriarchal spatial division of social life in rural areas. The nature of hostel space, as policed and contested by the South African state and the hostel dwellers themselves, marks a hitherto unexplored set of spatial relations within the apartheid city.

Using Massey's progressive sense of place, the hostel becomes a node in a web of meaning. This when we examine the microspatial relations of hostel ing and connections cut across gender lines and apartheid to reveal that the hostel—as a place—reverberates with meaning sectors of the South African population, not only the male worker legally inhabit(ed) its environs.

Which Elements of the Identity Debate Can Inform a Retheorization of the Hostel?

In examining the meaning of identity associated with hostels, we need a thorough understanding of which aspect of identity informs the inquiry and how identity, in turn, is shaped by the hostel. The analysis laid out here is not an examination of identity generally, it is specifically an examination of the intersection of race, sexuality, and gender. Within the growing number of theories that examine the links between race and gender, feminist authors like Gayatri Chakravorty Spivak (1987) and cultural theorists like Said (1993) have argued for the need to reexamine frameworks of identity. In *Yearnings: Race, Gender, and Cultural Politics*, bell hooks forcefully shows through language that, in the absence of an "appropriate sexual discourse," breaking the silence about the sexualization of black bodies, gender, and race is all but impossible without transgression:

> Sexuality has always provided gendered metaphors for colonization. Free countries equated with free men, domination with castration, the loss of manhood, and rape—the terrorist act re-enacting the drama of conquest, as men of the dominating group sexually violate the bodies of women who are among the dominated. The intent of this act was to continuously remind dominated men of their loss of power; rape was a gesture of symbolic castration. Dominated men are made powerless (i.e., impotent) over and over again as the women they would have had the right to possess, to control, to assert power over, to dominate, to fuck, are fucked and fucked over by the dominating victorious male group. (1991, 57)

Race Matters that "the con-
ates is rooted in visceral feel-
al myths of black women and
nt myths that inform the con-
women and men either as threat-
for sexual power over whites or
ite culture. Abdul JanMohamed
uss the interlinkages between race,
patriarchal history of sexual viola-
aster's rape of the female slave was
nowledge could not be admitted to in
ursivity lest it undermine the socio-
acial] border, which was of course es-
politica.   racism" (1992, 104). By exploring the
sential to the very su.
interlinkages between race, gender, and sex we begin to destabilize the
foundations of the racial myth. White fantasies about race purity are real-
izable only once the threatening power of the black body has been symbolically reconfigured as controlled, punished, and broken or as a passive,
de-sexualized parody.

The recent theoretical work on sexuality, gender, and race has sought
to show how race as a constructed category is informed historically by
traits that are signified in sexual terms. The particular way in which the
practice of racialization operates, however, is context specific and hints
at the importance of spatial relations operating on a variety of scales.

Patricia McFadden, a political economist working in gender studies
in sub-Saharan Africa, argues that "in the southern African context sexuality is central to understanding the reproductive, social, economic, political, cultural and religious roles we play as women and men" (1992,
165). She contends that female sexuality, and the resulting gender identities in all human societies, is constructed in relation to perceived male
pleasure and reproduction. The result of this externally constructed sexuality is that women are sexually molded as young women, wives, lovers,
or mothers. These labels, echoing apartheid's designated roles, McFadden
argues, are fundamentally restrictive to women because they restrict and
control the expression of sexuality, and therefore the women's potential
to occupy social, economic, and political roles. Very rarely is female sexu-

ality expressed in terms that do not revolve around reproduction or male pleasure. In the case of the hostels—specifically in the panoptic, albeit patently inefficient, glare of the state through local administrators and patriarchal elders and kinfolk—women found their lives and bodies objectified in ways that supported the heteropatriarchal dictates of apartheid's procreational economy.

Judith Butler (1990) has famously suggested that identity is a process of "performed signification" acted out by, and upon, the body. Identity, in Butler's terms, is not constituted by the physical body (object) alone. Rather identity is reformulated as a mediated result in the process of signification, which is constructed by society and acted upon by society in terms that the individual has some power to negotiate. For Butler, identity is neither the result of an overdetermined structure (like apartheid) nor the consequence of a biologically determined destiny (like sex). Instead identity formation is more fluid. Butler challenges the idea of a foundationalist subject identity, not the practice of assuming subject positions and representing oneself. Agency is not denied; it is simply reformulated as variations within regulated and habitual processes. Seeing identity as a process of signification acted out by and upon the sexualized body allows us to move beyond the idea of vacuous individuals "filled" by socially constructed identities, thereby restoring agency and subjectivity, without falling into the trap of biologically determined destinies.

Shireen Hassim and Lindy Stiebel (1993) used a similar notion of signification in their analysis of gender representations in South African violence. Using semiotic analysis, they show how black women in South Africa are typically depicted as, and naturalized into, passive roles, such as those of refugees. Hassim and Stiebel's work shows how the identity of black women—as signified by their actions, clothing, and bodily positions—is interpreted or acted upon as passive by the media in its portrayal of black "refugee" women. Hassim and Stiebel, however, fail to recognize that many women do not in fact passively accept the identity that they are assigned. For many women, the act of moving from one place to another is an act of defiance and a renegotiation of a subjectivity that has been sexualized *for* them under heterospatial conditions of the procreational economy of apartheid. Moving on from Hassim and Stiebel's insight requires that we examine both the portrayal of subjects (in Hassim and

Stiebel's case effected by the media) *and* the development of personal subjectivity that is performed by individuals themselves.

How or why is this theoretical insight useful for research on hostels? By way of illustration, the following critique, now more than thirty years old, of the "sordid" hostel system (a critique that continues to echo today in contemporary South Africa) demonstrates the extent to which hostel space was explicitly linked to sexuality, thereby reproducing a particular vision of patriarchal heterosexuality:

> In their plight to satisfy their sexual needs, [migrants] indulge in terrible practices such as homosexualism, which is an outside practice and is now beginning to reach broader extents. Young men reaching the mines get involved in this practice. There are even men (I am not exaggerating) who move around the compounds and their sole business is to entice men in the compound [or hostel] to sleep with them. Some men would even divorce their wives afterwards because of this practice that has become important in their lives. All kinds of atrocious vices take place in these hostels such as sodomy and the like. A close investigation of this problem would unearth quite a number of vices which are unknown to the public but common talk to the inmates of a hostel. (Mohlabe 1970, 4; quoted in Wilson 1972)

Instead of indulging the reader's fantastic voyeurism, Mohlabe could have focused on the deplorable conditions of hostel environments, the injustice of low-wage labor, and a host of other hostel problems. The critic describes the hostel in terms that relate specifically to the sexual subjectivities of the hostel population. Furthermore, the issue of agency and blame is directed away from the apartheid state and toward the "natural" needs of hostel men who have been "corrupted" by the system. Moodie (1994), Harries (1990), and Achmat (1993) have begun to unlock part of the role that sexuality played in the hostel system, although none has looked at the spatiality of that process.

Hostels served as a space of sexual anxiety for critics of the system. Same-sex desire articulated at a local and small-scale level, however, did not necessarily challenge the national-scale politics of heteropatriarchal desire and responsibility, connecting the lives of male hostel dwellers and their female partners and relatives. Both Harries (1990) and Moodie (1994) show that throughout the twentieth century, so-called *situational homosexuality* helped to shore up heteropatriarchal power for most men. The sexual landscape of the hostel defined women who had been spatially separated from their husbands in reproductive terms as obedient wives, mothers, and domestic homemakers. Women who refused to recognize the sexualized spatial boundaries and moved into the hostel during apartheid, became the focus of state-inspired moral censure because they were defined in sexual terms that were opposite to "the good wife." Critics and state administrators alike viewed women living in hostels as prostitutes and therefore out of bounds. Hostels operated as places that helped to deny black female desire and served the regime of spatial control by rendering their desire "illicit," thereby curbing its threatening capacity to bear children. Anecdotal evidence provided by women during the Truth and Reconciliation Commission's hearings graphically highlights how denigrating the black female body and its reproductive capacity was central to the operation of apartheid. This menacing fear, hidden in the subconscious of apartheid's practitioners and guardians, emerged with horrific and sometimes lethal results. The following account was provided by a black South African woman who resisted apartheid policy and was interrogated by secret security policemen:

> The other one came to me . . . and said, "Stand up! I want to see your vagina," and they started hitting me with fists. After that, they electrocuted us. . . . I can't remember where did they apply this to my body because, when they switched it on, I felt as if my private parts were falling. . . . While [I was] crying, they were sitting in front of me laughing. (South Africa 1998, ch. 10, 55)

Rupturing moments such as these suggest that for many women their bodies were literally war zones demarcated by a malevolent state. Those bodies (and men's too) were also incorporated into the hostel system to create the heterospatial conditions that would aid capital and an anxiously racist state.

A further reason why the sexual dimension of the hostel is important is found within the debate about race, gender, and sexuality. JanMohamed (1992) has argued that racialized sexual identities are predicated on the fracturing, rather than the unity, of the "black family." This involves the destruction of the paternal and maternal function within the enslaved family: the continued feminization of the black male, which is simultaneously symbolic and material and the convoluted masculinization of the black woman. Bell hooks concurs and extends JanMohamed's remarks (made with respect to the United States) to the South African context: "It is no accident that the South African apartheid regime systematically attacks and destroys black efforts to construct homeplace, however tenuous that small private reality where black women and men can renew their spirits and recover themselves" (1991, 46).

While both JanMohamed and hooks assert that the destruction of the black family is central to the reproduction of racism, their aspatial analyses cannot appreciate the ways in which heterosexual desires strung out over space and time held families together in ways that were sometimes simultaneously oppressive and resistant. In other words, the procreational geography of apartheid in South Africa was a spatial strategy to ameliorate the economic cost of complete black familial destruction in the interest of capital. The hostel is part of that regime of spatial control. It serves as a space central to the rearticulation of black family life into an economically efficient heteropatriarchal unit, extended over national space and time. This rearticulated heteropatriarchal unit differed from previous familial organizations because it was regulated at a national scale, unlike the regulation of heteropatriarchal family life prior to apartheid, which was more localized in extent and scale. The hostel as a significant spatial expression of apartheid was also part of the construction, control, and regulation of a sexualized racism.

What begins to emerge is a view of the family, and the differently sexed body within the family, as a fundamental site of struggle in the negotiation of raced and gendered identities. Holding onto the process-oriented notion of place outlined by Massey (1993), we need to examine how the situated subjectivities of individuals were sexualized and how bodies became objectified. Why were male sexualities constructed within the hostel, by the state and social critics alike, in terms that did not relate to their families, while female subjectivities in rural areas remained constructed in terms that related entirely to male pleasure and reproduction? The only possible explanation lies in examining how these processes were in fact mutually constituted, contradictory, and overdetermined.

New questions about migration emerge when we focus on the mutually constituted way in which sexuality and spatial location (the hostel and the rural home) regulated the flow of a gendered migration system. Migration becomes more than the consequences of economic pushes and pulls; it is the result of an apartheid system that sought to control the work of men and women in specific spheres.

How Does a Synthesis of Place and Signified Identity Inform the Existing Hostel Debate?

The debate surrounding identity formation has taken as its point of departure that identity is a negotiated process. Stuart Hall, for example, has argued that "identity is neither continuous nor continuously interrupted but constantly framed between the simultaneous vectors of similarity, continuity, and difference" (1990; cited in Chabram and Fregoso 1990, 206).

These similarities, continuities, and differences are also *spatialized*, and the hostel space is deeply implicated in that process. By looking at the hostel as an unbounded space in terms of the meaning it has for those associated with it, we emphasize linkages with the rural areas, the township, and a myriad of other geographical nodes. These connections are important because they illuminate how people living in hostels understand themselves and how others, in turn, understand them.

Given that the apartheid regime sought to restructure the black family household and reshape gender identity, what follows is an attempt to show how hostels were part of that destruction but also a locale where familial destruction was resisted. By adding to Massey's progressive exposition (1993) of "place" as a signified notion of identity, at least three windows open from which we can both view and revise the extant literature on migration and hostels: nonstatic identities, nonstatic space, and hostels as family spaces.

Nonstatic Identities

A nonstatic framework of the hostel allows us to examine it as a site of apartheid oppression and resistance simultaneously. At the same time, it

allows us to see individuals who participated in hostel life, directly or indirectly, as active resisters and not the passive victims of apartheid urban
planning; indeed, we can maintain a sense of these particular people as
subjects in their own right. Furthermore, following Butler—that is, viewing identity as an act of signification—also allows the researcher greater
freedom to examine the resistance of hostel dwellers. When we view
identity as a process of signification (both acted out and acted upon) and
continually renegotiated in the hostel context, competing identities become possible. For example, an economically and socially powerful black
woman is also a refugee, a rural mother living in an urban location, and
an illegal hostel tenant: "I am now an old woman. I have a house. My
children have respect for me. But here, here I am nothing. Here they do
not care if I am hungry, they do not even give me bread. Why would they
ask what I think?"[2]

Studies of the migrant labor system have tended to ignore gender relations, gender identity, and the role of women completely. Exceptions
focus on the sufferings of women without men or on the destructive social impacts of migrant labor—once again focusing on the particularity
of female experiences, usually within the rural areas exclusively. Within
these studies there is a tendency to subsume women within the family and
to privilege kinship at the expense of other social networks and relationships (Brown 1983; Sharp and Spiegel 1990; van der Vliet 1991; Naanen
1991; Parpart 1986). These texts often lack either a temporal or a spatial
perspective. A static notion of tradition is reified, and the apparent surface continuity in institutions such as the family, bridewealth, marriage,
and even migration obscures significant temporal and spatial differences,
leaving women solely the passive victims of patriarchy and apartheid. Even
findings from South Africa's Truth and Reconciliation Commission, docu-
menting how women were victims of apartheid, tends to locate the pain
and suffering of some women within a static atemporal and aspatial heterosexual matrix. Accounts by widows, now childless mothers, "groom-
less" brides, and fatherless daughters somehow render their tellers all the
more passive.

An exception to these generalized accounts concerning hostels is the
sustained work by Moodie (1988, 1992) that has demonstrated the ways
in which changing migration patterns in South Africa have yielded a

highly gendered migrant labor result. Moodie (1994) has demonstrated how changing migration patterns have molded and shaped emergent gender relations, particularly around issues like sexuality. The aim here is to advance these insights by examining men and women in contexts that are physically distant from their daily life but intimately involved in the processes of identity and self-identification. By focusing on the interconnections in this way, women in particular become active survival strategists, not merely apartheid victims.

Nonstatic Space

When place is viewed as a process and as nonstatic (Massey 1993), the hostel becomes more than a physically bounded space. Underscoring the extended notion of hostels, we also come to a closer understanding of hostels as so much more than batteries of masculine labor. Rather we are permitted a view of the hostel as a subjective space extending beyond its physical walls. With regard to identity, then, the identity-laden tentacles of apartheid that were shaped by the hostel experience extend into the rural areas and onto the bodies of family members thousands of miles away from the hostel. Many women found their activities shaped by identities that were not necessarily constructed only in terms of their immediate environment but rather in terms that related to places and processes hundreds of miles away. By refocusing the analytical gaze in this way, the hostel's significance and the identities that resulted from the hostel process come into focus as more than a physical urban place but also an important node within the network of heteropatriarchal identity formation. Related to that, the migration process (for *both* men and women) becomes more than a physical movement, but also an exercise in challenging—or at the very least responding to—the shifting meanings that the hostel as a place occupied within the family.

   Although the issue of hostels has received extensive attention from scholars, very seldom has the hostel been seen to extend into areas that lie outside its physical structures. Political economists, social historians, sociologists, and urban geographers have crafted rich accounts of contemporary and historical migrant worker life in cities. The alienating, exploitative, and inhumane condition of this apparently exclusively masculine urban lifestyle has been widely documented (Burawoy 1972; Gordon 1977; Keenan 1981; Laburn and McNamara 1980; Lipton 1980; Payze and Keith 1993). As part of the migrant workers' urban life, the heavily guarded hostel or compound also received extensive empirical geographical documentation (see Pirie and da Silva 1986; Crush 1992). While historical studies of hostels have demonstrated the changing nature of hostel spaces over time (Moroney 1978; Turrell 1984; Mabin 1986; Pirie 1991; Wentzel 1993), a static male-based ethnic focus has emerged with regard to hostel dwellers and their associated identities (Beinart 1987; Breckenridge 1990).

The collective point made by these authors is of a history of static rural-based ethnic identity, exacerbated by the ethnically segregated hostels that worked against the development of class consciousness. More recently, the crisis surrounding hostels and ethnic loyalties crystallizing into political affiliation raised questions surrounding the future of hostels (Crush and James 1991; Brookes 1991; de Kock et al. 1993), but offered no clue as to the reasons behind the convergence of ethnic and political identities. Current explanations for hostel dwellers' resistance to family housing, for example, can be located within researchers' adherence to notions of static rural ethnic identities (see Zulu 1993).

A static theoretical context framed the *Goldstone Hostels Report,* commissioned by the South African government. The report both qualitatively and quantitatively examined hostel life as an isolated experience. Titled *Communities in Isolation,* the report does acknowledge, among other facts, that the hostel never was a homogenous population and that, before upgrading can take place, the "complexity" of the hostel community must be understood (Minaar 1993). An ongoing subtext throughout the report tells the story of women living in hostels. Because the hostel is seen as an isolated space, it is impossible for the authors of the report to show how women are an integral part of hostel life. By physically sealing off the hostel in this way, they analytically close themselves off to the important elements of hostel life that can be understood only by viewing the relations between the hostel and other spheres. Examples of this approach can be seen in several in-depth case studies of hostel violence (Zulu 1993; Shaw 1993; Rubenstein 1993; Jones 1993). In *A Bed Called Home*

(1993), Ramphele shifts the "all-male" focus on hostels toward a more nuanced and complex set of gendered spatial relations.

Hostels as Part of Family Life

Ramphele (1993) in an exceptional way demonstrates how migration was an exclusively male institution. A focus on women also serves to break down the neat production/reproduction division that characterizes current accounts of migrant labor. Colin Murray (1981) and Walker (1991) have painstakingly shown how, in the face of declining remittances from migrants, rural reserves are increasingly becoming the sites of rural production. Similarly, Moodie (1980, 1992), Ramphele (1986, 1993), and Pamela Reynolds (1988) have shown that women are central to urban migrant work both as workers and, in their roles as wives and girlfriends, as support for male migrant workers. Also Bozzoli (1991) and Miranda Miles (1993) have documented, via oral testimonies told to them, the movements of women toward Johannesburg in the early twentieth century. Karen Jochelson, Monyaola Mothielei, and Jean-Patrick Leger (1991) have also clearly shown why the role of women must be addressed, as the migrant worker population totters on the edge of the AIDS precipice (see also Sher et al. 1981; Brink, Sher, and Clausen 1986; Hunt 1989).

Gendered migration studies have begun to unravel the complicated weave of identity that marked the apartheid era. Furthermore, this work has also set about showing how this process of gendering was in fact central to the operation of apartheid. Less well developed is the spatiality implicit in these debates. By nature, migration is a spatial process, but the exact way in which identity is affected by that spatiality remains unexamined.

Conclusion

The theoretical framework was sketched out to reinterpret the lives and families associated with hostel spaces across space and through time. As a spatial construct, the apartheid hostel is also an example of how racial exploitations occur through the regulation of sexuality and how spatial processes like migration are shaped by that experience. As a geographer, I am interested in how place and identity are intertwined. Further, I seek to show that the confluence of identity and place have material consequences for the lives caught up in the process and finally that the process is particularly gendered and "sexed."

The concrete nature of the apartheid legacy in the shape of the urban form needs reformulation, as do static understandings of identity. The theoretical framework described and developed in this chapter aims, in part, to do that. A signified sexual identity is shown to be negotiated in several ways that include a spatial dimension. As part of that process, a nonstatic sense of place also shapes that sexual signification. Because we have chosen to examine the particular ways in which race and gender are involved in the process, it is essential to examine how identity is linked to the sexualized body as the sign. The actions, or "signs," of those interviewed for the project are viewed as responses to identities that result from constraints—for example, a heteropatriarchal household structure that is shaped by an apartheid legacy. By extending our analysis of the household to include the hostel, we come to see how both men and women find their actions shaped by their subjective understandings as racialized and sexualized objects as well as racialized and sexualized subjects. The interplay of these two processes, which are different sides of the same coin, shapes the theoretical understanding of identity. That process of subjectivization and objectification is linked to the shifting meaning of places within the procreational geography of apartheid.

Throughout the study, and running parallel to a story of women's survival, is a second narrative. In the context of contemporary South Africa, survival still involves the incessant negotiation of personal and spatial meaning. Just as gender and racial identities shift in response to the demands of daily life, so too does meaning surrounding hostel space. In theoretical terms, when the signification of the hostels can mutate to absorb these changes, the status quo remains intact. When the negotiation of personal identity radically challenges the spatial meaning, a hostel crisis emerges.

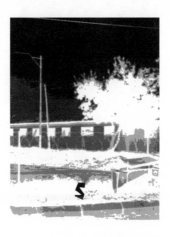

ΠΑΤΙΟΠΑL BALLETS

The continuous flow of men and women to and from European [read: white] centers of employment is one of the outstanding features . . . in the life of Native peoples inhabiting Southern Africa.

—Isaac Schapera, *Migrant Labor and Tribal Life*

SCHAPERA'S GENDERED and preapartheid comments provide an interesting contrast to current understandings of migration in South Africa. Today, half a century later, most scholars who are interested in South African migration patterns do not acknowledge that women continued to migrate and work as domestics or as illegal urban immigrants after the imposition of influx control policies during the apartheid era (1948–94).[1] By the late 1970s a static sense of identity and space had come to inform conceptualizations of migrant labor. Shula Marks and Elaine Unterhalter, for example, have argued that migration "has not only meant the oscillation of the male worker between his family and work place, but has also led to a very particular relationship being set up between women as the reproducers and subsidisers of the labour force in the countryside" (1978, 1).

This quote demonstrates the extent to which the apartheid state had not only literally divided up the landscape and labor, but had also influenced the epistemological framework used to understand migration. Like others participating in the debate about migration during the 1960s and 1970s, Marks and Unterhalter did not question the gendered division of labor and space. The concept of men as producers and women as reproducers was taken for granted as a point of departure for these analyses. Building upon a heteronormative worldview, these studies focused on the creation of a black laboring class through a Marxist production-reproduction framework. Operating within what Butler (1990) has referred to as a heterosexual matrix, classic works such as these ignore both the politics of gender and heterosexuality as it relates to migration. What Marks and Unterhalter (and others) failed to appreciate was that, while apartheid policy did shift the gendered dynamics of migration in South Africa, these changes were brought by imposing, in national space, a certain model of heteropatriarchy. At times this heteropatriarchy reinforced preexisting relations in South Africa, but in some cases it contradicted and even supplanted these preexisting models of heteropatriarchy in rural South Africa.

Marks and Unterhalter (1978) and others have argued that the apartheid objective was to locate male workers at the site of urban production and tie women to rural locales of reproduction. These functionalist perspectives showed that productive male labor in urban areas and reproductive female labor in rural areas were constituent parts in an intricate machinery of labor exploitation and racial capitalist accumulation. Admittedly, they were. But imagining productive male labor only in urban areas and reproductive female labor only in rural areas does not adequately reflect the lives of those caught up in migration in South Africa under apartheid or now. As we now know and as this work shows, women did migrate to urban areas and continue to do so. By contrast, some men remained in rural homesteads and continue to do so. At best, these men were lumped into a catchall reserve-labor army, while migrant women were designated as either male appendages or loose in every sense of the word. In all cases, these individuals were seen as aberrations to the broader political economy of apartheid.

In fact, as this research will show, most women (and presumably men) moved through periods of mobility and stasis. To assume that work and monetary value flowed only from mobile men is simply not true. Women worked in urban areas and rural areas; women made money in both places too. Indeed, it was sometimes women's rural work and remittances that supported men's stays and lives in urban hostels.

Andrè Leliveld (for example) has argued that, even after apartheid ended,

> With the wife bound to the homestead because of the children, temporary labor migration . . . is a feasible option for the husband to earn a relatively high income compared with activities in agriculture or (rural) industry. This money can be used to support the family and for savings that can be invested in future enterprises. As the wife usually does not generate income other than that from subsistence agriculture, the remittances have to be considerable and frequent to ensure homestead survival. (1997, 1843)

What Leliveld and others fail to comprehend is the intrinsic value of women's labor (formal and informal), or their mobility for that matter. These accounts do correctly assert that it is men who more often, and most visibly, migrate. However, we should not lose sight of the empirically grounded fact that an elastic family structure throughout rural South Africa meant that many women were able to migrate (perhaps not formally) by relying on other women or rural relatives to undertake child care for them while they were away. Indeed, the devaluing of women's work by Allan Low, for example, is astounding: "[I]n the prevailing wage employment market in southern Africa, young, educated and adult male members have the best off-farm prospects. It will thus be the older, less well-educated and female members of the household who are left to do most of the farm work. This will have a negative impact on farm production and the productivity per worker per hectare" (1986, 1845). South African feminist scholars have implicitly and explicitly critiqued that framework (Bozzoli 1991; Jochelson 1995; Miles 1993; Ramphele 1993; Sinclair 1998; Walker 1995; for an international collection on migration, gender, and geography, see Fairhurst, Booysen, and Hattingh 1997). Across this landscape, a network of relational ties and bonds between people (framed by heterosexual desire or responsibility) ensured that labor was reproduced in the cheapest way possible. This set of ties and bonds of desire differed from previous heteropatriarchal household systems in that the latter system stretched the household to a national scale. It is also through this web of meaning that most women migrated so as to secure the survival of their families. The conventional accounts of migration do not ask how and to what end the migrant labor economy of apartheid relied on a very particular heterosexual vision of family cast on the national scale. In so doing, the symbolic and practical politics of a particular kind of racialized heterosexuality promulgated through apartheid's heterospatiality remains hidden. Also, the survival strategies employed by many women who stepped outside either the conventional roles of childrearing or the conventional domain of the household (or both) remain hidden too and untheorized. Conventional tropes that use the division of labor and space as a context for explaining how migrant labor was pushed and pulled across the country argue that male migrant workers left rural reserves (the site of reproduction) for urban centers (or sites of production), where formal wage work was available. Invariably, these analyses have examined men and women as independent entities and not as the subjects of an interrelated family life.

These understandings have failed to come to grips with the desires and experiences of women. Quite simply, many women have stepped outside their designated heteropatriarchal roles as mothers and tenders of the home fires. These transgressions were not always undertaken as acts of defiance but usually for necessary and "mundane" reasons like feeding and keeping their families together. For women who migrated, the geography of labor was always more complex. More often, women migrated via nested and interconnected personal networks, as the following migrant woman's account reveals: "I come here to KwaThema for three months to sell the clothes I made and also to brew beer here in the hostel. This way my mother can look after my children at home and look after the chicken eggs business in Msinga."[2] Like the migrant work experience of men, many women also moved across the country, but their reasons for moving were more often related to their involvement in informal "home-girl" networks that had the combined effects of turning domestic work like cooking, washing, and beer brewing into paid employment when women relocated into settings away from their families. For the women who remained behind, remittances from migrating women ensured that household responsibilities were met, that children of migrant women were minded, fed, clothed, and that aging relatives were cared for.

When women migrated via networks of support, those movements took place upon and through the procreational geography of apartheid. Because women, within that system, were expected to mother, their mobility and movements were curtailed not only by stringent influx control policies, but by the real and symbolic demands of any one of the repertoire of heteropatriarchal roles fashioned under apartheid: sister, mother, wife, daughter. In this way, on the national landscape, men and women migrants participated in a delicate ballet of mutually supported acts of mobility. However, for women the balancing of domestic responsibility and mobility was more complex: it involved establishing a set of informal, usually women-dominated, networks of support. Reciprocity and mutual economic support defined many of these arrangements. By contrast, men's migration patterns remained nested in a set of support networks defined through heteropatriarchal relationships with their families and a formal economic relationship with employers or with the state, or both.

Within the web of heteropatriarchal responsibility and desire, women could not simply migrate if they wished to do so. When women moved, they upset the procreational economy: in moving away from the homestead, married women in particular shifted the locus of heteropatriarchal desire. They also loosened the place-specific lure of home space for male migrants.

Moving usually resulted in migrant women undertaking domestic work, either for white urban households or for male migrant workers living in urban hostels. While domestic work for white families and black men resulted in different life experiences, both arrangements secured support in the form of money, accommodation, or both. The work that women undertook before and after relocation differed from the formal wage work–related moves of male migrants.

South African feminist accounts have begun to document a fluid and ever changing relationship between women and work under apartheid and beyond. Feminist scholars have shown that, as both active migrants and rural homestead managers, women operate within a less rigid understanding of work and space. The complexity of their experience stands in stark contrast to the "reproductive" roles described by class-based analyses that have argued that women, who were not formally employed, were simply part of the industrial reserve army.

Adding to insights gained from feminist studies, this chapter will show how place-based experiences shaped by heteropatriarchy are important to understand the relationship between migrant women, their "work," and their decision to relocate. We shall focus on the experiences of women who have moved from the Msinga valley in KwaZulu-Natal and are living in the KwaThema hostel on the Witwatersrand in Gauteng. Those situated experiences shape identity and are explained as "the focus of a distinct mixture of wider and more local social relations and, further again that the juxtaposition of these relations may produce effects that would not have happened otherwise" (Massey 1993, 68). A woman KwaThema hostel resident described that relational web in the following terms: "I am here [in the hostel] because my *son* lives here. I am here because they burned my shack in KwaThema. I am here because I am a *woman without relatives* in Msinga. My *husband* is dead. What else can a *widow* do?"[3] Evidence from the interview shows how mobility and place are understood in terms of the place-specific heterosexual relationships the woman hostel dweller does or does not possess. Her movements are the resultant vectors of those subjective experiences of place. The discussion of heterosexual identity that flows from these mutually situated accounts does not simply reflect static, place-based experiences but also the way in which those processes are linked across space. By rethinking migration as a mutually situated account, we can transcend a traditional push-pull migration model that predicates a production-reproduction framework. Life histories show that migration is a spatial process informed by heterosexual meaning, not only an economic decision that has spatial consequences.

The dynamic process of place-based identity formation is further illustrated through two life histories. By seeking to strike a balance between income-generating activities (like beer brewing) and care-providing work (like mothering), women negotiate and challenge the heteropatriarchal constraints and opportunities that are presented by competing notions of place. Put another way, women migrate (or move between places), because the gendered politics of places present competing opportunities and constraints for women. Those opportunities and constraints are negotiated by way of identities circumscribed by heteropatriarchy.

Sex, Gender, and Migration: A Review

Women of Phokeng: Consciousness, Life Strategy and Migrancy in South Africa, 1900–1983 by South African sociologist Belinda Bozzoli (1991) is a celebrated account of women and migration. Using a life history approach, with the aid of researcher Mmantho Nkotsoe, she unlocks the broad processes and events that shaped the experiences of twenty-two black women born in and around Phokeng, in the western Transvaal. Bozzoli describes the domestic work experiences of these women in the white suburbs of early Johannesburg and their return to Phokeng, where she interviewed them just before the abolition of influx control regulations. Bozzoli shows how these women's recollections disrupt current conceptions of migrant workers held by academics and policymakers. She argues that the process is far more complex than traditionally held notions lead us to believe:

> These young women were both willfully independent, and caught up in the expectations of both the rural and the urban social institutions in which they were involved. Their consciousness reveals their desire to portray themselves as free agents, seeking to make sense of, and give cultural meaning to their experiences, but also shows their awareness that their efforts were shaped and sometimes thwarted by the demands of their rural families, their own sense of duty, and the requirements of urban employers. It is not easy to characterise these women either as collaborators in their own oppression . . . or resisters against it. It would seem that the actual, historically constructed consciousness is too complex to be forced into either of these two mutually exclusive categories. (104)

While the work rejects any easy categorization of women's lives, it works from a static understanding of place: "This focus on one particular village has a number of advantages. The women form a 'cohort' who convey narratives that spring from a common landscape, allowing us to identify with greater precision the mainsprings of the common and diverging patterns of consciousness each displays, and to give a thicker description of meaning and culture" (241). Bozzoli's "common landscape" is a departure point for her understanding of the development of consciousness. While a shared environment does provide a context for studying these women as a group, it does not illustrate spatial relationships of those lives.

Despite Bozzoli's at times aggressive insistence on the primacy of her respondents' words in shaping the analysis, *Women of Phokeng* is an interpretation, as Walker (1992) rightly observes. Bozzoli's epistemological claim about her relationship to her research subjects is stunning in light of her contention (in a footnote) that "feminist studies tend to suffer from this lack of contextualization, . . . [and from] the 'no history' romantic and populist approach, . . . in which it is naively assumed that an untheorised 'uncovering' of the words and experiences of women is possible" (274, n3). Notwithstanding the fact that her overgeneralized interpretation of feminist studies as untheorized is wrong (or at least outdated), it is her underscoring of contextualization that requires further attention. Her interpretation of life in Phokeng is "contextualized" in a political economic history and a "common landscape." Bozzoli's interpretation posits the environment as lying outside and separate from the consciousness of women interviewed. It is my contention that the experience of context and environment are shaped by consciousness.

Studies of migrant women can be recast as investigations that underscore the importance of a geographical imagination and its role in the decision to relocate. From this perspective, a narrow definition of consciousness that does not explore the terms of relationships to places does not capture the complexity of migration. Even though the construction of place breaks through in the words of those interviewed in *Women of Phokeng* (e.g., "Yes my child, the Golden City [Johannesburg] is a place for whites" [204]), Bozzoli's interpretation works from unquestioned assumptions about the links between consciousness and environment. For Bozzoli, environment and consciousness are not mutually constituted. Rather, a static environment is experienced by all in the same way. Her assumption ignores individual subjective geographic imaginations that were not shared by all who moved from Phokeng.

A second and equally important insight to the work on identity and migration is *Going for Gold*. In this work Moodie focuses on the gender-segregated male migrant labor force in South Africa's gold mines. He states that his "analysis emphasizes the gender identities of these migrants as men and the complicated way in which their practice of integrity intersects with male and female gender roles on the mines and in the countryside" (1994, 3). He argues against the conventional belief that mine migrant culture for men was only an economic strategy to retain patriarchal proprietorship over rural homesteads, as argued by Philip Mayer (1980). Moodie advocates a complex reading of culture informed by both the social and the economic: "Cultures must be understood and analyzed as overlapping aggregations of beliefs and practices inscribed with implicit and explicit understandings about the exercise of power and situated within and dependent upon social networks and economic bases" (21). Using oral testimony once again, with the aid of researcher Vivienne Ndatshe, he shows how male and female migration are different sides of the same patriarchal coin. He argues that rural patriarchies are constituted by systems of prestige linked to conceptions of manhood for men and women. Under the changing material conditions that were brought about through apartheid, these conceptions of manhood changed. So as to guarantee men's continued patriarchal power, women were denied access in any form (including a conception of masculine power that older women mentioned) to dwindling political and material resources brought on by the apartheid state. Moodie uses the changing sexual practices of men and women as evidence of the changing patriarchal relations. The result is a nuanced and complex story about the development of "patriarchal tradition" under apartheid.

In keeping with Bozzoli's contention, Moodie shows the difficulty of categorizing the work of South African migrant women. In light of the "evolving" patriarchal tradition that is tied to material conditions in rural areas, female migration is explained as a necessary response: "[S]ome women achieved a 'male-dependent independence' which, while it paid lip service to traditional male rights, actually undercut the dominance of particular men over particular women. Others struggled to do double duty as both town women and country wives" (1994, 32). Interestingly, however, even Moodie appears to lack the vocabulary to describe these women as migrants. Their migrant mobilities are hidden in his naming of their identities (town women, country wives) in static, place-specific ways. Moodie also shows that a loss of access to workable land and a shortage of wage work for women meant that women became more dependent than ever on male relatives. As the system began to crumble for men, women found their access to land severely limited (through rural overcrowding, environmental degradation, and increased proletarianization). As a response women began moving to the urban areas because there was no possibility of male support in many areas (for another example of the process at work in colonial Rhodesia, see Schmidt 1991).

We can now extend Moodie's analysis of power and networks by demonstrating the extent to which those relations are implicitly and explicitly spatial. We need to extend his understanding of the material environment to include a subjective understanding of place. Place on the procreational geography of apartheid can be reflected through the lens of heterosexual desire, power, and responsibility. Movement on this landscape can be read, simultaneously, as moments of spatial foreclosure or opportune portals of mobility. On this landscape granted or denied mobility for bodies always depended on the symbolic heterosexual markings they exhibited. Thus, we can explore nonmaterial dimensions of migration, which include subjective experience.

In what follows, we see that place and identity are intimately tied by way of relationships configured in heterosexual ways. Further, and contrary to Bozzoli and Moodie, we see that the reasons behind a decision to migrate are not exclusively located within the realm of the material environment. Drawing on the descriptions of KwaThema and Msinga in chapter 2, here identity and place reverberate, collide, and coalesce in individual ways, thereby constructing a sense of place that is both a subjective and an objective experience. That experience of place, in turn, informs a decision to migrate or remain in place. Second, heterosexual identity and place are shown as mutually constructed in the two life stories that follow. By focusing upon lived experience in Msinga and KwaThema in this way, I hope to simultaneously create a strong case for place-based analyses of migration studies as well as a justification for locating sexuality at the center of the investigation of migration.

The relationship between identity and place can, of course, be examined from any number of different viewpoints. However, it is the contention of this work that the heteropatriarchal relations as configured during apartheid need attention in the present and for that reason heteropatriarchal framings of place will inform the analysis that follows.

Migration: Negotiating Place and Identity

For women, the negotiation of place can be understood at the household level. On this scale a complex negotiation of heteropatriarchal apartheid forces (like mobility) and household heteropatriarchal relations (which still include polygamy and bridewealth) merge, collide, and contradict.[4] Relationships between the heteropatriarchal household organization and the heteropatriarchal apartheid state are not fixed. In fact, the competing visions of heteropatriarchy lay at the heart of early struggles to impose an apartheid order. As Anne Mager and Gary Minkley argue in examining resistance to apartheid in East London in the 1950s,

> These conflicts brought out not only moral dissention between urban and migrant men, men and boys, migrant men and urban women, but also revealed the pressures on patriarchal relations in the community. While women defended their right to head independent households and make their own choices, their sons were hacking out a new path to manhood in hostile urban terrain and in the face of aggressive patriarchal resistance. If young men defended their mother's independence, they sought control over their girl-friends. (1993, 245)

However, even in their very insightful analysis, little explicit attention is paid to the unquestioning way in which the apartheid state imposed a patriarchal order that was also heterosexual. In the early 1950s apartheid legislation sought to change the household relations from those of a peasant economy to those that included sharecropping and ultimately proletarianization.[5] Later still, as apartheid reached a crisis, the relations within the heteropatriarchal household were once again contorted to achieve an apartheid ideal that took the form of homelands or "independent" states. In the late 1980s the heteropatriarchal household in Natal and the apartheid state engaged again and what emerged was an ethnopatriarchal "reality" that served to undermine the progress of the national liberation movement (for a detailed discussion see chapter 6, as well as Waetjen 1999; Hassim 1993; Hassim and Stiebel 1993). This time, however, Inkatha (with the apartheid state's support, as recent findings by the Truth and Reconciliation Commission have shown) encouraged an antagonistic ethnic-based position in opposition to growing ANC resistance and wide-ranging support. Party leader Buthelezi articulated the terms of Inkatha's ethnoheteropatriarchy: "When God Almighty gave the female species the most onerous task of human reproduction, He in His divine wisdom had assessed the human qualities of women, before He made the decision that it was you our womanfolk, and not us men who would perform the task with bravery under even the worst conditions which we blacks have to endure even within as oppressive a system as that which existed in South Africa" (quoted in Waetjen 1999, 674). Clearly, the words of Buthelezi underscore the fact that in the construction of a Zulu nationalism, the role of gender was uppermost in his mind. However, it is also worth repeating that the vision of gender that he described operates within the confines of the procreational economy of apartheid. Not once, for example, did Buthelezi ever suggest that women leave their rural homes and defy the influx control laws that supposedly held them in place.

Within the dynamic relationship between the heteropatriarchal apartheid state and the black heteropatriarchal household, women have always had to balance the demands for income with the responsibilities of human reproduction. The balance of these weights (income provision and heterosexual reproduction and child care) defined women's work. For women living in Msinga, movement between places is the spatial negotiation of this balance.

In the past and under apartheid laws like influx control, women also confronted the apartheid state directly. Since the end of apartheid and in contemporary South Africa, however, the heteropatriarchal legacy of apartheid and the household struggles around heteropatriarchy continue: women still negotiate income *and* care provision. As part of the balancing of survival, the organization of household space is central. For example, the echoing of the rural homestead in the reorganization of hostels on the inside cannot be explained without appreciating the linkages between both places. Identical beer-brewing rooms in both places, within ear- and eyeshot of common food preparation and child care rooms in rural KwaZulu-Natal and urban KwaThema, are one way in which we see how domestic responsibility and income-generating activities are balanced by women's networks in and across space.

A fundamental difference, however, lies in the way in which women's work in the form of beer brewing within that spatial organization is interpreted in a place-specific way. In Msinga the task is undertaken without remuneration, while brewing in KwaThema results in financial income. By exploring this link we begin to see that, by migrating, women negotiate the household politics of survival and responsibility by relocating. The precise origin and destination of that relocation, however, is evidence of a geographic imagination that is based not only in a material reality. Indeed, decisions to move draw on imagined and subjective experience of place.

Drawing on the insights provided by the extant literature on women and migration in southern Africa and a sense of place as sketched out above, we now turn to the events, circumstances, and lives of the particular migrant women living in the hostel in KwaThema. By underscoring an extended notion of hostels, we also come to a closer understanding of South African hostels today as more than pools of masculine labor. Rather, we are permitted a view of the hostel, both historically and in contemporary South Africa, as subjective and gendered and heterosexualized spaces extending beyond the barbed-wire fences. This view, however, takes on meaning only when tied to place-based histories, personal experiences of residents living in the hostel and their connections to other places like Msinga, KwaZulu-Natal.

With regard to identity, then, the apartheid tentacles on the scale of national organization extend via local spaces like the hostel and the home area and into the lives of family members miles apart. For women interviewed in the study, these tentacles defy an understanding that relies solely on a racialized explanation. Rather, women become involved in the hostel system through their heterosexual identities as wives or mothers. The migrant identity (for men *and* women) becomes more than a physical movement, but also an exercise in challenging, or at the very least responding to, the shifting meanings that the KwaThema hostel and Msinga present as places both materially and as subjective experiences.

Negotiating Placed Identity

The placed experience of violence in KwaThema and Msinga demonstrates how the perceived and real fear of heteropatriarchal political violence can shape places. To date, work focusing on migration among women has collectively shown how the decision to migrate is made within the constraints of a patriarchal order. In all cases, the women interviewed for this study stated that the decision was shaped by relations with a male individual like a husband, brother, father, or uncle. In this regard this work is not exceptional. What I will add to that understanding, however, is a perception of movement as a response to the heteropatriarchal demands of the place.

As a result of the ongoing violence, many of the women interviewed here have lost the male relatives who represent the relational link to a heteropatriarchal order. However, the death of a male relative does not necessarily mean that a woman is free of the bonds of heteropatriarchy. Rather, the multiple scales at which this insidious system operates, guarantees that women without husbands still operate within a world and by way of a spectrum of identities shaped by the place-specific and multi-layered politics of heteropatriarchy. Because of ongoing violence in their home region, many women have also lost the support of a male patron. As fatherless, widowed, or abandoned mothers, many of the women interviewed in this study moved within an established female network of support. And while it is clear that these networks are historically rooted in a rural heteropatriarchal order, with time these same networks have taken on a shape that grants some women freedoms within the renegotiated spatial confines of the hostel. For example, by relocating to hostels women can charge for applying their domestic skills. By remaining in rural Msinga women cannot renegotiate the terms of their social position. By relocating to the hostel and through the income generated from informal work there, women living in the hostel can, at the very least, negotiate an identity in a less rigid social space and in turn survive.

Part of negotiation of survival requires a move to another place invested with historical and contemporary meaning. The hostel embodies that place for the women of Msinga. The hostel is by no means free of heteropatriarchal systems of control, but it does present a viable economic and social opportunity for women who have in some sense fallen between the cracks of a traditional, albeit shifting, domestic heteropatriarchy.

The negotiation of survival by women is a situated process. Negotiating the gendered identity of mother, female business partner, or girlfriend, women cultivate, co-opt, and resist identities that are mutually constituted by both the KwaThema hostel and the Msinga region. It is also worth noting that these identities are not exclusive at any one time, or over a life period, but represent a continuum of experience and negotiation of identity undertaken by women in relation to hostel space.

MOTHERING

Of the thirty women I interviewed, twenty-two had children under the age of twelve. As mothers, these women argued their maternal identities had resulted in their move to the hostel, where they were at least able to sell their domestic skills in return for cash. One respondent showed how mothering presented a spatial tension. She had moved to the hostel and away from her children in order to reinterpret her domestic beer-brewing skills into paid work: "My children are part of my work decision and work life. They're why I'm here brewing beer, but when I am here I'm always worrying about them at home. . . . I'm their mother."[6] The elastic nature of household was amplified by another comment from a mother living in the KwaThema hostel. She, too, had come to interpret mothering as the act of providing for her children, even when it resulted in her physical displacement: "My eight kids need money. I manage to see them sometimes, but my role as their mother is to provide, and working here is one of the few places that I can do that."[7]

FEMALE PARTNER

The identities of the women I interviewed were also constructed in terms that extended beyond the sphere of mothering. Still, within the confines of patriarchal expectation and power, the new arrivals and other women who had lived in the hostel for almost four years stated that negotiating access to the hostel space was in some instances through a male connection: "My boyfriend lived here before me. I need to check things with him

—like when I moved into the hostel—he arranged it for me, but now that I am here it's not that important when I run the business, but I still like to check stuff with him."[8] The spatial tensions and constraints involved in negotiating a heteropatriarchal web in both Msinga and the KwaThema hostel that lead to a decision to move into the hostel were further underscored by the following statement: "I came to KwaThema after mourning for the five years after my husband was murdered in Msinga. I needed to create an income. In Tonado [an informal settlement] I met my boyfriend, who arranged for me to live here. Now I sell beer to his hostel friends."[9] Physical cultural constraints, like the traditional mourning period in the last case had resulted in the financial ruin of the respondent. After five years, her decision to move to the hostel proved successful only after her close association with a male hostel dweller resulted in the economic viability of her beer-brewing venture.

Unlike the first wave of women to settle the hostel community some three years before, a second wave of women who relied on those established networks told life stories that were connected to the hostel and the associated female-dominated domestic economy: "I live here through my sister. Her and her husband originally rented the room. As her sister she invited me to help out with the beer business that she runs. As my own business was not going that well I moved in here, as the rent was cheap."[10] A further example demonstrated that these arrangements were part of a wider set of female-dominated networks that had emerged in Msinga more recently: "Through my mother's friend I sublet this room. My financial problems at home were too great. Now that my children are here with me, I can look after them and earn an income."[11]

These quotes suggest the hostel is a space to which women have migrated because it provides a context in which their identity can be temporarily reinterpreted. Still operating within the confines of heteropatriarchal constraints, like widowhood, and gaining access to hostel space, most of the women interviewed demonstrated how living in the KwaThema hostel provided the economic means whereby they could mother their children, who are often located in Msinga, more than three hundred miles away.

As mentioned earlier, for most women interviewed, daily life and life-long histories tell of how their identities are constantly renegotiated and reinterpreted. The two life stories that follow show how these identities come together throughout a life.[12] The two cases, on a practical level also show the two phases of migration evident in the hostel: women who were pioneers, and "second" generation migrants who take advantage of the migration chain already in place.

Case History One

Khonzapphi Qwabe is a forty-five-year-old self-described widow, mother, and beer brewer. Her migratory life history reveals a household struggle for survival that resulted in thirty years of oscillatory migration between the Msinga valley and KwaThema. Since the late 1980s moving to survive has taken on a meaning that extends well beyond its economic dimension. Mounting violence in Msinga and KwaThema has threatened her life on more than one occasion.

Khonzapphi, unlike many other women in the KwaThema hostel, has chosen to maintain a strict Zulu dress code at all times because of her Zulu beer clientele. Every day she wears a light-brown herbal face paste and darkens her facial scars with soot. Within the urban context of Kwa-Thema, this dress code was a clear signifier of her Zulu status. Her movements between Msinga and KwaThema began in 1963. She balanced beer brewing for money in KwaThema with returning to Msinga for the births of her three children, the deaths of relatives and two children, and for harvesting, caring for aging relatives, and, more recently, attending political rallies in KwaZulu. Although she learned brewing from her mother, she recalled that her mother had not moved between rural and urban areas: "It is woman's work to brew beer. Lucky for us, you can brew anywhere. The recipe is here [pointing to her head]. . . . As long as my memory is good and my body is strong, I'm fine." She explained how she discovered as a young woman that beer brewing was easily transferable from her rural home, where she brewed it as part of her rural responsibilities as wife, mother, and daughter. After a short visit to Kwa-Thema three decades ago, she learned from a friend how it was possible in the urban areas to earn money from beer brewing. Since that time, she had balanced her life between these two domains.

Balancing income and responsibility changed dramatically for Khonzapphi in 1989. Unknown gunmen in the KwaThema hostel murdered her husband, whom she had married when she was eighteen. Until that point,

Khonzapphi had always resided in the informal settlement of Tonado, a short distance from the hostel, during her urban visits. Widowed, without a formal tie to Msinga, and in the face of rising anti-Zulu sentiment in the township, Khonzapphi became an easy target for malicious acts of vandalism and theft in the informal settlement. All this escalated until early one morning she awoke to the sound of neighbors' yells. Her shack had been set alight: "One night I awoke to hear screaming and shouting. I went outside. The settlement where I lived was in flames. People were running everywhere. There was only one [water] tap. It was a terrifying night. I was no longer welcome there." Like most of the single Zulu women in Tonado, she had been violently evicted by individuals who had earlier attempted to burn down the hostel a short distance away. Along with the eighty or so other women, she decided to move into the hostel, which had also been badly damaged during a week of township carnage. Her eldest surviving son, himself an illegal, unemployed hostel dweller, arranged for her temporary stay.

When the interview took place, Khonzapphi stated that she would probably continue to sell beer in the hostel. Missing from her comment, however, was any recognition of the need to balance care and income. Instead she spoke of a suspended relation to both places: "I live between both places now. . . . I belong to no place. I have no husband in Msinga, I have no husband here—only a son, but it is not the same." She no longer sees herself as a migrant. Her husband's family had relied on the income of their murdered son and cannot offer support to her—their widowed daughter-in-law. Khonzapphi clings to the hostel through her son's tenuous status. By losing claim to Msinga and her social roots there, because of her husband's death, she has little choice but to move away.

Case History Two

Disesile Shange is a twenty-six-year-old Zulu woman and mother of three. Two of her children (aged seven and eight) still attend school in Msinga while the third currently lives with an older friend in Soweto, some thirty miles to the west.

Disesile's migration pattern spans close to twelve years. Her first visit to the Vaal area was to visit her sick father, a migrant worker living in a hostel in Benoni. As a young girl she nursed him back to health and about a year later she returned to Msinga: "I was the youngest daughter. I was not needed at home as much. Also, it would be a while before I was going to marry and so my mother sent me to look after my father. He was sick for a year. I lived in a room in the township. I worked for that family to pay for the rent, and then cared for my father there too. When he got better, I left." Back home, she stayed in her family's household until she married a childhood friend. Soon after the marriage, she moved out of her family's home and set up her own house close by. During the first few months her husband attempted to grow crops to support himself and his wife. It soon became apparent to both Disesile and her husband that one of them would have to move into the formal wage market in order to survive: "After two years of failed crops, there was no money. Life was getting hard and another child was expected. There was no choice but to look for work away from Msinga. First my husband, then me."

In 1987 her husband came to KwaThema to look for work. Over the next three years he failed to secure permanent employment. In order to supplement their household income, Disesile decided to leave her children with her mother and visit a sister who was also living in KwaThema. During this visit she learned from her sister that selling services like beer brewing could make income: "Things were easier for a while. We both tried to make a living here in KwaThema. No work, just odd jobs here, and a little money to send back to my mother for the children. But this place is bad. It killed my husband. The tokoloshe is here."

After the murder of her husband in Msinga in 1989 and during a five-year mourning period, Disesile decided to move away from Msinga in the hope of finding support for herself and her children. Somewhat ambiguously, she went on: "The time of mourning was very bad for my kids. I was not allowed to seek work. I had to stay at Msinga. There is no work there. The time of mourning keeps you in your place."

After the financially ruinous five-year period required for mourning (experienced by close to one third of the women interviewed), however, she decided to follow her sister to the urban area on a more permanent basis. By that time her sister was already living in the KwaThema hostel. Later the sister moved into the township. Disesile's presence had allowed the sister to move out of the hostel and at the same time secure and build on their beer market niche. When Disesile returned home, her sister moved back into the hostel and ensured that their informal beer-brewing business continued to operate.

Disesile pooled her income with that of her sister, who was connected to the hostel, even though she had moved into the township. They both supported children who lived with their grandmother in Msinga. She described her status as a widow in the urban areas as one that tended to make her life difficult, as she was always "in the way," although at home she did not encounter this social awkwardness: "The choices for a widow are slim. There is no support from anyone. Life is a struggle. I rely on my sister here [KwaThema] and my mother at home [Msinga]. Its different when there is a husband. There is his family too; they will support you. But now its just my kids, my sister, my mother, and me."

Conclusion

While the creation of places through networks and networks through places is at the heart of understanding identity and its migratory consequences, we should not romanticize this process at any level. Living within the hostel and these networks is a problematic engagement for all women. As more and more women are drawn into the hostel, competition increases and beer prices drop. As the providers of increasingly cheaper beer, these women inadvertently increase the levels of alcoholism among the under- or unemployed hostel community. Furthermore, the constant abuse of alcohol also feeds into the ever widening vortex of public and private violence that defines much of hostel life.

Nevertheless, at a household level women under heteropatriarchal constraints have managed to eke out existences (see figs. 5.1–5.2). Despite the contradiction that alcohol production presents, the geometries that extend from and toward nodal places in the real and imagined South African landscape lie at the center of the decision to migrate. Often, the decision to migrate is not the active undertaking that much of the literature suggests. For the women interviewed in this study, migration is a subtle process of negotiation through time and space, a process that finally results in the permanent or semipermanent displacement of individuals

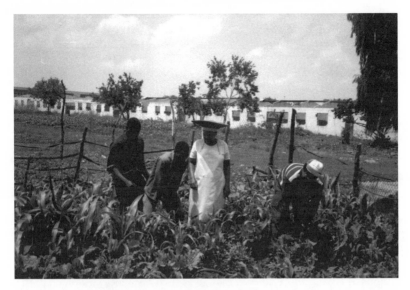

Fig. 5.1. Woman hostel dweller overseeing agricultural activity inside the hostel yard. The men in the picture are unemployed hostel residents who worked in return for beer.

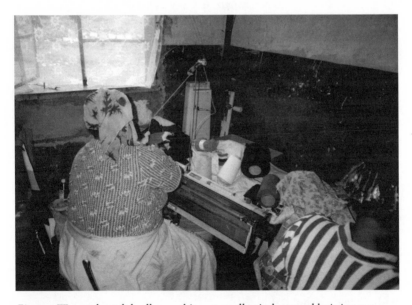

Fig. 5.2. Women hostel dweller working at a collectively owned knitting machine. Clothing was made for personal use and sold in an informal trading store close to the hostel gate.

from one place to another. In other African contexts and without the extensive spatiality reflected here, networks of support between poor women have been referred to as economies of affection (Hyden 1983). When economies of affection extend over space, these informal economic geographies also provide networks (informed by subjective experiences of place) that become women's decisions to migrate, or not. It is of the social capital caught up in these networks that David Webster hints: "Male dominance is gained in the most alienating of experiences, for migrancy generally means living and working with strangers in hostels and factories in a hostile environment. Their womenfolk have a different set of experiences. Their relationships are crafted communally, in socially rewarding circumstances, such as work parties or shellfish harvesting expeditions. It is this, above all else, that gives such resilience to women in the domestic struggle" (1991, 268). It is not surprising, then, to discover too that these networks become the backbone of women's migratory patterns.

Interestingly, the direct impacts of apartheid, while clearly shaping the lives of black South Africans at a national level, are hidden on a more personal scale through heteropatriarchally defined gender relations. As wives, daughters, and mothers, the women who migrated to the hostel in KwaThema did so in order to fulfill responsibilities resulting from their identities within a wider heteropatriarchal context.

The internalization of these identities, and the accordant spatial movement, is also a process that occurs between two or more places and flows in both directions. The movement to the hostel at KwaThema from Msinga is also tied to the internalized way in which individuals understand the spatial geography of the South African landscape. Learning to read the procreational geography for survival is a skill passed on and developed by the women interviewed. Different places provide very different opportunities and constraints.

The preceding description and analysis reveals that the effects of apartheid are nuanced and inscribed onto the bodies of individuals through sexed and raced classification. The process by which apartheid set about discriminating between and within "race" groups is tied to a gendering within the household.

As the reality of this situation is brought to bear on the current transformative effort in South Africa, questions remain about how policymakers can reverse how apartheid influences continue to operate. One way is by the reconfiguring of the real and symbolic meaning of specific spaces like hostels. Simply removing restrictions upon movement through- out South Africa does little to relieve the topography of difference that was, and still is, deeply etched onto the physical and mental landscape. The preceding analysis has attempted to show that, as the women inter- viewed have come to read, interpret, and balance opportunity and adver- sity in places, so too must those interested in changing the system learn to read the heteropatriarchal landscape of contemporary South Africa.

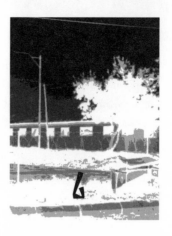

A MENACING TRADITION

> Never in its history has South Africa been subjected to such high levels of political conflict as has been the case for the past twenty years. Despite the significant socio-political changes that have taken place in the last three years and the various efforts to reduce the conflict, the levels of conflict and violence continue to be unacceptably high.
>
> Much of the conflict has been concentrated within black communities and an important recurring feature has been the conflict that has developed between hostel residents and members of the surrounding communities. This has frequently resulted in some of the most violent incidents South Africa has witnessed. As a result, many have come to view the hostels as a key problem within the much larger context of protracted violence in South Africa.
>
> —Justice Olivier, *Communities in Isolation*

IN 1993 THE GOLDSTONE Commission of Inquiry regarding the Prevention of Public Violence and Intimidation presented a collection of findings about hostel violence (Minnaar 1993). The findings included quantitative and qualitative research that sought to uncover the causes of violent antagonisms between people living in migrant worker hostels and people living in communities outside the hostel walls, in the township at large. The above quote opens the findings of the collaborative research project; a grave tone suggests hostel violence in South Africa has a long history and that the causes lie in the broader context of political violence in that country. Given this opening, the irony of the study's title, *Communities in Isolation,* should not escape a curious reader: why are hostels and those who live in them consistently viewed as hermetically sealed off from the "real world" when their condition is tied to the broader political and social context? This paradox, born of heteropatriarchal theories of South African society, plagues work about hostels, hostel dwellers, and hostel violence.

The official study failed to present the "hostel community" as anything less than a cohesive, homogenous social unit. While the official study admitted differences *between* hostels, it did not examine differences *within* hostels. Disappointing but not surprising, the account omitted the increasing numbers of women who had moved into hostels throughout the region from 1985 onward. Because no mention was made of the gendered nature of hostel transformation, the contested politics of heteropatriarchy also escaped attention in the Minnaar report (1993), an oversight also evident in more general accounts about hostel violence.

While the actual numbers of women who moved into hostels throughout the region are impossible to estimate, Lauren Segal (1991), Sitas (1996), and Mamdani (1996) all mention the presence of women in hostels. The mere mention of women, however, does not inform a more thorough analysis of the gendered dynamic within hostels at the time. The presence or absence of figures, however, does not preclude us from conducting an analysis that locates gender and sex at the center of the debate about violence in hostels between 1990 and 1995.

Violence is always gendered and the lacuna about women hostel dwellers also meant that accounts about violence were nongendered. Missing is an analysis that seeks to examine the ways in which a masculinized violent form of heterosexual power was challenged and reasserted during this time. Hints of this struggle are reflected in the newspaper accounts and rumors of female rape, female assault, domestic abuse of female

family members, and acts of violence undertaken in the interests of pre-
serving heteropatriarchal visions of family. We also see how policy debates around the conversion of hostels into family housing was interpreted
by male hostel dwellers as an effort to undermine their claims to turf. The
result was a violent reaction that, among other factors already well elucidated by others, was also an attempt to hold onto apartheid's heterospatiality.

While most studies suggest that ethnic nationalism and economic impoverishment colluded to create an isolated and stereotyped community of
male hostel dwellers in the East Rand townships of the early 1990s, these
findings emerge because the scale of the research highlighted struggles
between "hostel dwellers" and the "township community" only. What the
findings failed to show was how the hostel community itself was a deeply
divided, always gendered, shifting, and transient group of people. *Communities in Isolation* and studies like it employ the intransigent apartheid
architecture of hostel and township as the epistemological model through
which hostel violence is understood. The arguments operated within an
implicit spatial understanding of tensions between hostel versus township and the belief that violence diffuses spatially from the hostel to the
township. By employing an alternative framework that sees the hostel as
a nonstatic space, like the hostel dwellers interviewed we too can understand the hostel as located within interconnected geometries of power
and relationships between far-flung "homes" and the hostels.

Because previous studies have employed a static notion of community, their accounts of hostel violence were most noticeably nongendered.
Despite sensational newspaper accounts about female rapes in hostels
(*City Press*, 2/16/92; *Vrye Weekblad*, 4/8/92) the heteropatriarchal face of
hostel violence has escaped attention. Instead, authors and researchers
examined the hostel as a static ethnic space, cut off from the world.
Newspaper accounts of violence against women worked on the assumption that women close to or living in the hostel deserved their fate; they
were at the wrong place at the wrong time. But of course hostels are neither disconnected, nor nongendered spaces. The hostel is deeply implicated and felt in the lives of family members who live hundreds of miles
away, but also by the many who circulate between its walls and their rural
"homes," not least of all by the women who undertake that journey.

Weaving through the Goldstone Commission's findings are hints that the violence between hostel dwellers and the citizens of the townships in which they are located may be the result of male hostel dwellers' fears of a diminishing patriarchal authority, not in the hostel per se but in rural patriarchal households. A survey of 750 male hostel dwellers living in fifteen geographically dispersed hostels found that it was in fact plausible that the majority of hostel dwellers living in the most violence-prone hostels (53%) favored retaining the single-sex hostel system (de Kock et al. 1993). Further, it was shown that the most violence-prone hostel dwellers in the study strongly objected to the presence of wives and children, or any system that would create such a set of circumstances. In fact, half the entire sample (men living in both violence-prone and non-violence-prone hostels) argued that the presence of families in hostels would signal an end to their ties to rural homesteads and, by association, the power they wielded in those settings. However, the implications of these findings were not expanded upon. Instead the "male hostel dweller" was held up as the legitimate bed holder and therefore entitled hostel resident. Ironically, *his* "legitimacy" was defined by the then crumbling illegitimate and now debunked apartheid order.

Despite the astoundingly high proportion of male hostel dwellers who clearly saw the retention of hostel space as a means by which they could hold onto dwindling rural-based heteropatriarchal power structures, the authors of most studies on hostel violence failed to examine the question of masculinity, or gender, in any way. Indeed, *Communities in Isolation* and the studies contained in it operated within the heterosexual matrix that has defined much work on migrancy in South Africa. Nowhere is the heteropatriarchal assumption more evident than in the words of the authors describing their research methodology: "The fieldwork was executed by young, but experienced and properly trained black female workers. . . . Previous fieldwork in hostels . . . revealed that young ladies were best able to establish rapport with hostel residents" (de Kock et al. 1993, 176).

Let us take a moment to investigate how this methodological statement biased the research undertaken and how the results of this project could not possibly have revealed anything but a reinscription of heteropatriarchal desire and power. As feminist theorists have convincingly shown, the identity of the researcher does in fact shape the results (Finch

1984; Lather 1988; Cotteril 1992; Edwards 1990; with respect to southern Africa, see Miles and Crush 1993). However, what makes this unabashedly sexist research methodology particularly egregious is that women interviewers presumably were used as a lure in a highly contested heteropatriarchal context. Although the "ladies" hopefully came to no harm while conducting the fieldwork for this project, we can assume that their encounters with hostel dwellers were nonetheless tinged with hues of heterosexual interaction; in fact the research could be construed as a "bait and switch" exercise! Unlike the work of Dunbar Moodie, for example, which has consistently employed the findings of Vivienne Ndatshe (see Moodie 1994) in a self-conscious and purposeful way to uncover the complexity of migrant masculinity in Pondoland, the work of this state-sponsored research undertaking concluded, unsurprisingly, that proper control should be exercised over the "illegal" residents in hostels. Presumably, many of those "illegal" residents were women.

We begin by examining the Goldstone Commission because of its importance in the debate about hostel violence in South Africa, but also because the report reveals the perils of imagining the "hostel community" as a unit. The Goldstone Commission, and in this it is not exceptional, also draws on apartheid-inspired and deeply gendered definitions of legality and illegality, thereby legitimating the claims of a diminishing number of formally employed and registered male hostel dwellers. However, studies of hostels and violence since the publication of this landmark study have deepened our understanding of "the hostel community." In fact Segal (1991), Sitas (1996), and Mamdani (1996) stand out as exceptionally nuanced examinations of the alienation experienced by hostel dwellers. Notwithstanding the contribution of even these works, when scholars frame their analysis of who is inside or outside the community in nongendered terms, they inadvertently draw on apartheid-inspired notions of legitimacy.

Hostels and Ethnicity

The reason why the idea of the hostel community is so pervasive in contemporary work on hostels is because life in hostels is viewed in unproblematized heteronormative and patriarchal terms (exceptions include

Ramphele 1986, 1989a, 1989b, 1993). This literature has nonetheless made a significant contribution to our understanding of ethnic nationalism, economic restructuring, and labor in South Africa by way of an ethnic lens (e.g., Breckinbridge 1990; Sitas 1985). In so doing, authors have shown how networks of workers from rural South Africa fostered relationships in hostels that were often explained by way of hierarchies, gerontocracies, and associations at home.

From the middle of the 1980s, however, work on the ethnic makeup of migrant worker hostels and compounds located on the Witwatersrand, or in the region today known as Gauteng, tended to focus on the rise of ethnic nationalism. Specifically, work has paid attention to the rise of ethnic Zulu nationalism through the machinations of power that emanated from the Inkatha Freedom Party (IFP). From the mid-1980s onward, the IFP "ideologically negotiated the weighty legacy of a century of territorial and social partitioning that belied claims of a unified 'Zulu nation'" (Waetjen 1999, 661; but see also Hassim and Stiebel 1993; Adam and Moodley 1992; Campbell, Mare, and Walker 1995). Interestingly, these more recent accounts (and the interviews conducted for this project) contrast markedly with the deeply gendered ethnic identities documented by Webster (1991) in the coastal Kosi Bay district of northeastern KwaZulu-Natal. From the mid-1970s and throughout the 1980s, Webster notes that private rural domestic spaces, in some parts of KwaZulu, created a social context within which women's identities differed significantly from those of their migrating male relatives: "In this case they are exacerbated by the strains exerted on relationships by the wrenching experience of migrant labour. Placed alongside this is a conundrum: why do the men of the area espouse a 'Zulu' identity, while women cling to a 'Thonga' one?" (1991, 266).

With the self-evident collapse of the apartheid state in the late 1980s, however, a reassertion of male "Zuluness" throughout the area of KwaZulu ensured that gender became one of the battlefields whereupon ethnic identity was fought. For over a decade now, commentators have argued and shown how a cauldron of Zulu nationalism was tended closely by former homeland leader and present-day cabinet minister Mangosuthu Buthelezi. Notwithstanding the charismatic—some might argue egomaniacal—vision set forth by Buthelezi, the African National Congress did outmaneuver the IFP in the 1980s. While the stranglehold of apartheid lost its grip in the 1980s, the ANC made significant inroads into the urban black proletariat support base. The economic restructuring of capital resulted in the depopulation of hostels by traditional forms of labor (Crush and James 1991). Into these vacant spaces moved rural migrants. On the Witwatersrand, these migrants were most often from the area known today as KwaZulu-Natal. Indeed, as more and more women also began to migrate, the experiences and identity-forming spaces where those experiences took place changed too. Prior to this period it was argued that "Migrant labour separates men from women, and provides the means whereby men can strengthen their position of dominance. Migrancy is also the vehicle for the acquisition of knowledge of 'Zulu' custom and behavior, and the tools of the trade of women's oppression" (Webster 1991, 268). In the early 1990s, however, it became clear that this elegant heteropatriarchal division of space was under threat. Economic and political conditions made it necessary for women too to move into the vectors of Zulu identity formation; in geographical terms, women became migrants between KwaZulu and the Witwatersrand. Sitas (1996) and Mamdani (1996) provide a detailed mapping of part of this dynamic process within the hostel system. While almost silent on the role of women in this hostel repopulation process, these latter accounts do help to document what was also most certainly a gendered process.

In a work aptly titled "The New Tribalism: Hostels and Violence," Sitas (1996) argues that violence in hostels on the East Rand must be understood within the broader context in which hostel dwellers (migrants) are battling a process of marginalization. He traces, by way of a case study, how the men living in the Vosloorus hostel during the late 1980s were alienated from organized labor and evolving grassroots political movements in townships. However, while the trenchant analysis by Sitas does document the development of Zulu nationalism in the hostel system, the study operates within a heteropatriarchal epistemological framework. In other words, Sitas assumes that male hostel dwellers and their associative rural power structures (founded on normatized heterosexuality) are at the center of the debate about hostels and their future. Missing from his analysis is the insidious web of power that locates male hostel dwellers at the center of this debate and women at its margins.

Indeed, Sitas argues that the ethnic violence in hostels is the result of "alienation, disvaluation, disoralia and *degendering*" (emphasis mine), but his gendered analysis does not go far enough to uncover some of the other root causes of violence in the hostels. In his view, the process of alienation, disvaluation, disoralia, and degendering amounts to an assault on the male hostel dwellers' sense of self. Part of that assault on the self has resulted in "an aggressive regendering of male roles and patriarchal pride. . . . It is precisely crises within these cultural formations that create a climate of turbulence that in turn animates the rise of social movements." Sitas argues then that degendering amounts to "the pressure on gender roles as men and women are thrown into the mill and ground" (1996, 238). Fair enough. However, from the perspective that apartheid operated within a clearly understood and defined set of gender roles, for women in particular degendering is not necessarily an oppressive process, like alienation for example. Degendering is oppressive only if we valorize heteropatriarchal gender relations. For women and men, presumably, this degendering process is *gendered*. In other words, the effects of degendering are different for men and women. By failing to examine the gendered and sexed nature of this process, this work operates within the maze of heteropatriarchy. Nowhere is the peril of this viewpoint more telling than in Sitas's description of the process whereby hostels became "repopulated" by nontraditional residents:

> As *individuals* and *families* moved to the urban areas and specifically to the hostels, the vacant beds were taken up by a new kind of "migrating" *population* inside the hostels: *newcomers* who moved from bed to bed and from dormitory to dormitory. *People* who had been pushed off the land, despairing of waiting at the labour bureaux for jobs, without any "permit" to be in the areas, occupied the unoccupied spaces. . . . *This group of dispossessed people* did not necessarily "sponge off" others, however, but survived on temporary work provided by the industry in the area, or "relief" work provided by hostel inmates. (1996, 239; emphasis mine)

The sleight of hand in Sitas's argument occurs when he moves from a discussion of male hostel dwellers to this paragraph, wherein he admits to the presence of families in hostels. As the analysis continues new hostel dwellers become nongendered objects. Because no explicit mention is made of the changing gendered dynamics of hostels during this time, the male migrant hostel dweller and his subjective experiences become the standard by which legitimacy is measured. This male-centered analysis nevertheless draws, if unwittingly, on the heteropatriarchal framings of the apartheid state. The effect is one that masks the complicated gendering of hostel space that occurred at this time. In other words, when families replace male hostel dwellers, and in particular, when women replace men, the sexed and gendered geography of apartheid is challenged, and so too is the heteropatriarchal division of space and labor. Sitas ignores what I have referred to throughout as the procreational economic geography of apartheid: the many practical and symbolic ways in which South African men and women were expected to mother and father, and to unquestioningly assume the power relations that trickled out of that expectation and how those ways were regulated and contested in spatial terms. Men are always viewed as legitimate heads of households, entitled to urban shelter. By contrast, women in hostels are viewed as "transient," "visiting," or worse still, "looking for it." It is surprising that most studies fail to examine the change in the social makeup of the hostel population from a sex-gender perspective. Sitas points out that these new residents sometimes moved "from bed to bed" and while that is true, the consequences for women moving from bed to bed are quite different than they are for men. He also posits that this "group of dispossessed people" did not necessarily "sponge off" others. More than supporting themselves, if this group of new residents (and more especially the women) were similar to the women interviewed for this project, it is possible that "new" cohorts actually supported the lives of male hostel dwellers who were eking out existences in the formal, albeit shrinking, work sector outside the hostel.

In a work from the same year, Mamdani (1996) argues that a long historical view of the process reveals that the hostel dwellers at the center of this struggle were marked differently at different points in time. Highlighting the two decades that opened with the Durban strikes of 1972–73 and closed with the hostel-centered violence of the early 1990s on the Reef, he argues that a metonymic shift occurred regarding hostel dwellers. Whereas in the early 1990s hostel dwellers came to represent "rurality" in the urban, in the 1950s, for example, they were recognized as the cutting edge of antichief struggles in the countryside. Notwith-standing his nuanced tracing of how this came to be, like Sitas his analysis operates within an understanding that sees that shift in ungendered ways. A brief quote taken from his methodological field notes concerning in-terviews with hostel dwellers underscores this point:

> In the first half of 1993, I interviewed many of these, initially as part of a Durban-based COSATU (Congress of South African Trade Unions) research team charged with understanding the "needs of hostel dwellers." That effort bore little fruit. . . . With the assistance of a union organizer, I persisted for the next month, but little happened. I was able to meet with one male resident of Dalton Hostel and ten women living in Thokoza [women's] hostel. . . . I met the ten Thokoza women workers for several evenings of long conversations, as I did one organizer assigned to me. Eventually I realized the reason behind my difficulties. . . . A little discouraged, I moved to Johannesburg. (1996, 255–56)

Even after being indulged by ten women hostel dwellers, Mamdani does not note the significant ways in which these women's presence or insight might be important to his findings. Even discussion of "family housing" later on does not acknowledge that women migrants themselves might be considered legitimate consumers of upgraded or converted housing. In fact, when women or families feature in the argument, they do so as problems: "The problem was that the situation changed radically once influx control was abolished in 1986. The shanty population grew dra-matically. The more those hostel residents who wanted to live with their families moved into shanties, the greater was the likelihood that many of those remaining behind would also be exercising an option—for not liv-ing with families" (272).

Troubling is the erasure of women as hostel dwellers altogether. By arguing that women were surgically removed by "family" men into the shanty settlements fails to acknowledge that women continued to live out lives in hostels after 1986. Like Sitas, Mamdani views women migrants and hostel dwellers in ways that confine them to roles defined and dic-tated by the crumbling apartheid order.

The earlier but equally insightful work by Segal (1991) documents what she describes as "the human face of violence." By interviewing men living in Thokoza and Katlehong, she captures the process whereby people living in hostels perceive that they are under siege: "by the late 1980s . . . ethnicity was able to raise itself as a powerful force obscuring the commonality of working-class interests. The interviews suggest that gerontocratic rule persisted, home-based allegiances remained intact, and union-based associations were restricted to the factory floor" (1991, 206). It is into this vacuum that the IFP sought to mobilize an alienated cohort of mostly Zulu-identified migrants. However, even in Segal's work there is the suggestion that this change was also accompanied by a shifting in the gendered makeup of hostel life. One hostel dweller tells her, "more women started popping in. They would come and get water. . . . I didn't like it at all because a lot of women would stay and there would be a lot of corruption" (211). In light of these comments, Segal argues that, while women appeared to be moving into hostels, male residents were reluctant to speak about this issue. It is therefore perplexing why Segal did not seek out women hostel dwellers herself. Perhaps the heteropatriarchal trappings of the debate about hostels have blinded otherwise insightful analyses like Segal's from exploring the gendered aspects of hostel life. In fact, toward the end of her study, she mentions a struggle about women in the Thokoza hostel. However, the gendered aspects of hostel life remain unexplored by this otherwise excellent examination of the society of people living in hostels.

Sex, Gender, and Hostel Violence: The Case of KwaThema

With this critique in mind, we can examine the vortex of violence that shaped the lives of those who lived in the hostel that formed the basis of the research for this study. What follows here is a case study of one particular hostel during one protracted period of intense violence and bloodshed in KwaThema between 1990 and 1995.

During that time, the KwaThema hostel entered the national spotlight. More than anywhere else, events in the KwaThema hostel were used to exemplify a regional trend. The increasing numbers of Zulu hostel dwellers from KwaZulu who had moved into the PWV (Pretoria-Witwatersrand-Vereeniging) hostels were viewed as a marginal, but po-

Table 6.1. Political Affiliation of "Legal" (Male) Hostel Dwellers
and Surrounding Township Population, ca. 1991

Party Supported	Hostels (n=101)	Township (n=330)
Inkatha Freedom Party	71%	10%
African National Congress	12%	43%
National Party	7%	17%
Undecided	10%	30%

Source: Industrial Monitor 1993.

litically volatile, group (Reed 1994; Sitas 1996). Hostel and township
dwellers were shown to have widely differing experiences of places and
these experiences created differing political affiliations.

A considerable amount of material at the time and since has posited
ethnopolitical cleavages as the cause of hostel violence (see Table 6.1).
These ethnically focused analyses failed to recognize that, along with an
increasingly Zulu ethnic order in hostels, the sexual makeup of the hostel
population was also changing to include more "visible women." Even in
hostels where women were not residents, a heteropatriarchal vision held
sway. Furthermore, hostel dwellers and hostels in general came to represent the apar-theid state's homeland system for most that lived in the
township. Rather than hostel residents representing rurality, as Mamdani
suggests, in the early 1990s the hostel became a spatial metonym for
apartheid rurality. An apartheid history behind the creation of hostels
meant that when hostel dwellers made arguments in favor of retaining the
hostel system, their position was interpreted by the surrounding township community as one that favored a retention of the apartheid order.

It is important to note that, throughout the PWV region, discussion
about the hostel conversions galvanized *male* hostel residents' political
support for Inkatha. While Sitas's work posits economic reasons for the
alienation experienced by male hostel dwellers, we see here that a debate
about the future of hostels has in fact circulated in hostels and townships
since the mid-1980s and was instrumental in unsettling hostel dwellers:
the mere suggestion of hostel conversions upset a heteropatriarchal worldview and the procreational geography of apartheid.

Since late 1989, Inkatha, using KwaZulu as a regional base, had set about rallying political support throughout the country. In particular, they targeted an older, Zulu-speaking, and impoverished proletariat who had migrated from KwaZulu to the PWV in search of work. With the use of patriarchal imagery, like warring Zulu impis and Shaka's defeat of the British, Inkatha presented an adumbrated version of Zulu history that provided a "safe option" for older and fearful black male workers. For the growing number of Zulus who lived in the deteriorating hostels in the PWV, the sense of alienation was heightened as antiapartheid township politics raged and in some instances focused on the hostel as a symbol of apartheid. As a minority party in most East Rand townships, Inkatha came to articulate an increasingly appealing position for hostel dwellers that saw the hostel as home. Inkatha's sense of history imbued an idyllic rural past with a hierarchical cultural order where old age was respected and a "traditional" sexual division of responsibility prevailed. Inkatha leader Buthelezi, addressing a rally of women argued, "You are the women of Inkatha, begotten on the soil of South Africa, the daughters of Africa, you who begot the present generation and you through whom the nation will survive into the future are one of the great strengths of Inkatha. Ever since King Shaka laboured in this part of the world to create a nation, it is the womenfolk who have been custodians for so many" (Buthelezi, 8 October 1983, quoted in Hassim 1993, 17). The violence that followed in KwaThema and throughout the region had little to do with tradition; it was rather a direct result of Inkatha's culturally encoded struggle to assert a patriarchal order in the face of mounting political support for the ANC. The ANC had at this point, in part, paid lip service to ending the "traditional" oppression of women. Public attacks on entrenched institutions like polygamy, female circumcision, and bridewealth had begun to get attention (see Bazilli 1991). The patriarchal imperative surfaced with particular effect in the hostel. A KwaThema hostel dweller was reported as saying, "Six years ago it seemed the government had decided to phase out the single-sex hostel for some 700,000 migrant workers. . . . Although we were living as 'married bachelors' we made the best of the worst. We never expected anybody could influence us against one another in the hostel in this way" (*City Press*, 8/26/90). The quote reveals how the hostel conversions threatened a particular masculine identity: the married bachelor. The conversion debate was defined in such a way that the inclusion of women in upgrading schemes became the reason for much of the violence that followed, as male hostel dwellers fought for their status as "married bachelors." As married men living in the hostels throughout the PWV, these older Zulu migrant men could maintain a semblance of patriarchal power because the rural power base and access to land would remain intact. Once female relatives moved to the urban areas, however, control over the declining rural base and the accordant patriarchal social relations were threatened (for this argument with respect to male migrant miners, see Moodie 1994). It was not surprising when it was reported some time later, "Several thousand Natal Zulu hostel dwellers at a rally yesterday expressed their opposition to ending the single-sex hostel system in South Africa, saying they had not been consulted on the issue. . . . According to the speakers, it would be impossible to transform single-sex hostels into family units and accommodate all the present hostel dwellers and their families" (*Citizen*, 5/29/91). The English-speaking press continued to present the KwaThema hostel as a cauldron of seething ethnic rivalry. By using "essentialist" notions of Zulu identity, reports ignored the complexity of hostel-related social processes. Hostel violence was actually a highly gendered and local contestation for power linked to Inkatha's national political movement. Male hostel residents with established family networks extending across the country were represented as fearful of their future displacement, especially if the hostel was to be converted into family dwelling units (Schreiner 1991). As mentioned above, its is in this vortex of change that the IFP began its mobilizing efforts. As Segal (1991) argues, many hostel dwellers were in fact ignorant of the actual policies of the IFP. Indeed, most male hostel dwellers understood the IFP to be little more than a rallying cry for some kind of unity around a series of issues. Despite the often confused political implications of IFP policy, most IFP supporters seemed united in their desire to protect a vision of heteropatriarchal family life that had taken root during apartheid. Missing from these "genderless" debates were the accounts of women whose lives were connected to the hostel, as well as input from women who had already moved into the hostels.

In late 1990 then president Frederik Willem de Klerk, having released the jailed ANC leader Nelson Mandela earlier that year and eager to demonstrate a break with apartheid, spoke out against the single-sex hostel system. The migrant worker municipal hostels became the focus of a highly publicized media campaign during which de Klerk called for an end to single-sex hostels (*Beeld,* 8/30/90; *Natal Witness,* 8/29/90). Protracted national debate in the media injected new vigor into the hostel question. Violence in and around hostels continued to soar as male residents interpreted de Klerk's call as evidence of their future displacement by "families."

National Politics and the Design of "Family" Housing

By refocusing its efforts on hostel upgrading, the government had hoped to appease the material demands of hostel dwellers and thereby quell so-called hostel-related township violence. Results from *Communities in Isolation* argued that the government would be well advised to retain aspects of the single-sex hostel system. The proposal advocated a transitional model of hostel planning. It was recommended that the single-sex hostel should be superficially upgraded without any structural changes and that the same buildings would be transformed into family housing some time in the future (*Sunday Times,* 10/9/90). Echoing the earlier liberal critique of hostels, new proposals argued that by addressing the material needs of hostel dwellers and ultimately bringing families into the hostels, violence would cease, old-style apartheid would be scrapped, and family life would be restored.

The proposal did not acknowledge that families had always been part of the hostel and that some female-headed "families" had already moved into the hostels, preempting the official call. As a consequence to women living in hostels, postapartheid planning looked remarkably similar to planning during apartheid. Their informal work lives, which balanced income and household responsibility, were still devalued, and their links to hostels, regardless of how they were upgraded, were still dependent on male relatives. Although the nuclear family as a socioeconomic unit has seldom characterized the rural black family (van der Vliet 1991), suddenly it was argued that "Happiness is a home with his [male migrant's] family" (*Star,* 3/10/93).

At this time hostels were also undergoing a radical transformation in other parts of the country. Cape Town's hostels too were being slowly transformed into spaces that housed families (Ramphele 1993). Hostel transformation in the black townships of Cape Town, however, must be understood within the broader geography of apartheid and the highly differentiated way in which that policy was implemented between 1948 and 1994 (Smith 1992). An extreme housing shortage in Cape Town, tied to the racist employment policies enacted throughout the region during apartheid, forced families into crowded hostel spaces. These movements, however, did not precipitate the same violent reaction from male hostel dwellers. While I believe the differences between the experiences of Cape and East Rand hostel dwellers lies well beyond the scope of this chapter, the noted differences do underscore the complex and place-specific ways in which hostels as a spatial technology figure in the procreational economic geography of apartheid. "By the close of 1990 the recently unbanned African National Congress, the South African Communist Party, and the South African government established an alliance that set R4 billion [$1.2 billion at the time] aside for these conversions. To manage the funds an independent trust was established" (*Sunday Tribune,* 10/16/90; *Star,* 10/17/90).

Proposals soon followed: "For each family unit in the hostel, one has to move 15 people . . . to create facilities for the community, we recommended that the opportunity for small business be encouraged and that older disused buildings be used as workshops to generate self-employment. Hostel dwellers that were unemployed could be used as builders in modifying the hostels" (*Daily News,* 10/18/90). The findings of an unabashedly sexist architectural survey argued, among other things, "Three types of hostel dwellers were identified: The migrant worker who had invested in the homelands over a period of time and was not looking to settle in the city. Those with urban aspirations who could not afford to live in the township although they aspired to move and integrate with the community. Those men too insecure in their employment to think about integrating into the community argued that they planned to return home" (*Daily News,* 10/8/90).

A decade later, the definition of hostel dweller has changed little. Missing from these and even more contemporary insights, of course, are the visible and invisible hostel women; women who had been linked by association to hostels throughout their history, many of whom were already living in hostels. This gender-blind approach continued to define the hostel-upgrading question in local municipal policy documents, in the view of "representative" committees in the hostel, and finally in the way in which the issue came to be defined on a national scale.

Conclusion

By relocating the hostel and associated violence within a broader framework, the argument laid out here has sought to reimagine the ways in which violence in hostels during the 1990s affected men and women. Further, we see how violence in this context is a social process tied to the politics of femininity and masculinity in a society caught up in social change and the politics of transformation. Arguing that a crisis around the perceived erosion of heteromasculinity resulted in a period of protracted violence in hostels in the early 1990s does not detract from the contributions of others to this debate. Rather, what we see here is that violence is, in part, the result of a challenge to heteropatriarchy encoded on the apartheid landscape.

The notion of a homogenous hostel community is also incorrect for at least two reasons: First, people living in the hostels are not "isolated," as much of the policy literature, in particular, suggests. In fact, the lives of people living in hostels are deeply implicated in contiguous and farflung geographies. By examining these linkages within the context of a procreational economic geography, the different ways in which power circulates through these networks have been foregrounded. Second, the hostel is and always was a gendered community, and analyses that do not unpack the gendering of hostel space miss a great deal about the complex social systems that operate within their walls and connect them to the outside world. While some may counter that not all hostels experienced an invasion of women dwellers, as was the case in KwaThema, what we see here is that the presence of women does not preclude analyzing the hostel as a gendered space. As Moodie and Breckinridge have shown, hostels are places where masculinity and power are contested even without the presence of women.

By locating the hostel on the procreational geography of apartheid and seeing it as part of apartheid's heterospatiality, we are granted a new way of seeing contemporary hostel politics. First, the hostel is an interconnected node on the landscape. Its meaning extends well beyond its walls, and at times its symbolic meaning as a battery of masculine Zulu labor is more important than its reality: a fracturous, divided, sometimes chaotic, but always gendered population. Second, by examining the hostel as part of the procreational geography of apartheid, we are able to interpret the marginalization of women hostel dwellers from contemporary hostel conversion debates. Not least of all, the analysis laid out seeks to challenge historical racialized accounts of South Africa between 1948 and the present that fail to employ gender, sex, and space as analytical categories.

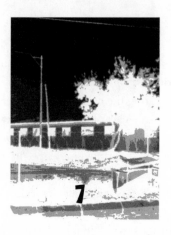

7

UNDESIGNING WOMEN

HOUSE, HOME, hearth. These three private spaces, when set alongside public spatial signifiers like factory, street, and bar, incite a gendered response. The warm, inviting, nurturing, and always feminine evocation of private spaces contrast markedly with the hostile, busy, noisy, always masculine associations of public space. Women are associated with and expected to operate within the context and confines of private space, while men and all things masculine articulate (and are articulated), control, and express in public. Public and private spaces, however, are mutually constituted. Put another way, there is no private space without public space, and vice versa. The policed division of space is particularly marked in heteropatriarchal societies, like apartheid South Africa's, and is in fact an integral division on the procreational landscape of both apartheid and contemporary South Africa. In societies such as these, the spatial dualism (public-private) operates in such a way that women are erased as active agents from the landscape. Often, their subjectivity is denied and they are channeled into spaces so as to reproduce the normative structures of heteropatriarchy: homes where they produce and rear children.

Informed by this feminist geographic imagination, we will examine the provision of housing in contemporary South Africa and, in particular the process whereby housing is delivered to those currently inhabiting old municipal hostels. Using a case study, this chapter shows how women (either as hostel dwellers or as wives in rural reserves), who were active creators of the conditions under which their families lived in hostels, are presently sidelined from contemporary hostel conversion discussions and debates. We will see that the marginalization of these women from the hostel-upgrading process occurs, not least of all, because heteronormative and deeply gendered ideas about legitimacy and stakeholders, informed by an apartheid past, shape policy in the present. Remember, the argument pertains even to those hostels where women are not present. Black South African women have always been part of the migration process and, by association, the hostel system. Whether actually present in contemporary hostels or not, the contributions of women who worked in and for families caught up in the hostel system (a process that extends across space and time) must inform debates about hostel conversion. They are legitimate stakeholders in the future of that system—whether it is retained in its current form, altered, or abolished.

The promise to provide adequate housing is an important component of contemporary politics in South Africa today. In the early days of the new South African administration, responsibility to provide housing fell to the Reconstruction and Development Program (RDP). For hostel dwellers, this program translated into bold plans to upgrade existing hostels or transform apartheid-designed hostels into postapartheid family housing. The hostel reconstruction project is one way in which the government plans to address the massive housing shortage in South Africa. The gendered lessons we can draw from it, while taken from an extreme context are, however, wide ranging and certainly applicable to other housing development projects throughout South Africa.

Throughout this study, the heteropatriarchal dimensions of hostel space have shaped my analysis. As the future of the hostel system is debated in South Africa, architectural designs show how hostels can be converted into family housing by moving women into hostel spaces (Dunstan 1992). It is male hostel dwellers that are consulted and form the core of participatory negotiating councils in hostels. Indeed, it is these same men who also worked, sometimes violently, to exclude women as active consumers of hostel housing. In short, the legitimacy enjoyed by these male hostel dwellers is, under the current dispensation, illegitimate.

It is surprising that few commentators have remarked on the lack of input from contemporary female hostel dwellers, or from women more generally. The exclusion of women from housing debates, while regrettable, is not unexpected. In a variety of settings throughout the world, the exclusion of women from debates about the use of space, and housing in particular, is well documented (Tinker and Summerfield 1999; Schlyter 1996; Gilroy and Woods 1994; Weisman 1994; Chauhan 1986).

Elizabeth Grosz has examined the interconnections between gender, sexuality, and the design of houses. She links the concept of architecture with the "phallocentric effacement of women and femininity" (1995, 47). In an examination of Luce Irigaray's reading of the history of philosophy, Grosz argues that the way in which space has been historically conceived of has always functioned either to contain or obliterate women. She goes on to argue that the enclosure or erasure of women from men's physical space is not unrelated to the containment of women in men's conceptual universe either. When we take Grosz's point and apply it to housing issues in South Africa, we see that, particularly in debates around "family housing," women's input has been obliterated. In its place, conventional tropes about women as nurturers, in accordance with the heteropatriarchal framings of apartheid, have informed debates.

The Economic Context for Housing in the New South Africa

To examine the gendered dimension of housing provision in South Africa, we need some understanding of the context within which the new government set itself the ambitious target of building one million homes between 1994 and 1999. After a brief review of housing policy since the new government came to power, we will also examine the gendered dimensions of the recently unveiled and controversial macroeconomic policy in South Africa. Within that context we are able to evaluate the case study of hostel upgrading in KwaThema.

Housing in Contemporary South Africa

In the RDP pamphlet that was distributed throughout the country after the 1994 elections in South Africa, the ANC government ranked housing, education, and a cessation of violence as its top three priorities. Later on in a government white paper entitled *A New Housing Policy and Strategy for South Africa,* the new government proposed the construction of one million houses between 1994 and 1999, to be paid for through a generous budgetary allocation (5 percent of the state budget). Housing advocates' hopes turned to doubt, however, when by 1999 the average allocations averaged closer to 1.5 percent for the previous five years. When compared with the largest allocations—22 percent for education and (quite oddly) 18 percent for defense and security—housing ranked only eighth on the list of government spending. Although the housing figures represent a significant increase when compared to the previous apartheid government's budget, the figures still reflect a small fraction of the proposed total spending.

From very early on, the new government has argued that, although housing will remain a priority, responsibility for its implementation will have to take place at the local and regional scale of government (for a policy statement, see Cobbett 1993). By implication, and because of the financial constraints imposed by the national housing budget, creative, cost-effective local initiatives will necessarily shape the character of future public housing in South Africa.

In a recent audit of the RDP, Bond and Khosa (1999, 10) caution that judging the implementation of the housing policy is less than straightforward. They argue that while it is clear that the national budgetary resources allocated never came close to those promised, actually counting the number of houses built between 1994 and 1999 is almost impossible because what constitutes a house remains debatable.

In an effort to aid the localized delivery of housing, in April 1996 the National Housing Finance Corporation was established, as well as the People's Housing Process, a government program focused on supporting self-help housing. The People's Housing Process provides homes for the very poor in South Africa, especially those who cannot afford traditional mortgage financing. The organization promotes local initiatives through the establishment of housing support centers throughout South Africa. It is at these support centers that the poor are given access to subsidies, serviced land, skills training, advice, building materials, and technical assistance.

Within this context, the two regions under study—Gauteng and KwaZulu Natal—combined make up close to 60 percent of the housing shortage in South Africa (SAIRR 1997, 757). It comes as no surprise then that within these two provincial contexts housing shortages are at crisis levels.

As part of that local-regional alliance, the productive utilization of hostel space is one initiative that has received wide-ranging support. As evidence, almost 15 percent of the proposed housing budget in 1994 was allocated throughout the ten regions for spending on hostel upgradings.[1]

For hostel dwellers and the families attached to them in KwaThema, housing has been delivered after extensive consultation with an apartheid-inspired definition of *hostel dwellers,* and has usually resulted in hostels being converted into a combination of upgraded single-sex and masculine accommodation, as well as family housing. None of these renovated schemes deliver housing to working women or to working mothers who are not part of a nuclear family. What is more disturbing is that this policy guarantees that the delivery of one of South Africa's rarest commodities —housing—is given to men more often than women.

Macroeconomic Policy in Contemporary South Africa

More recently, however, the RDP has been effectively sidelined and resituated as a program within the broader macroeconomic strategy that South Africa will pursue in the twenty-first century. Under this new dispensation, the Growth, Employment, and Redistribution macroeconomic policy (called GEAR), women's economic empowerment is not assured (Valodia 1998). Indeed, since it was first publicly announced, GEAR has been highly controversial, and it continues to be so. Some critics have argued that GEAR marks the government's break with the objectives of the RDP. They assert that GEAR is essentially a neoliberal economic strategy (see Adelzadeh 1996; Michie and Padayachee 1997). Others have argued that GEAR is consistent with the ANC leadership's positions on macroeconomic discipline, which were aired prior to the 1994 elections (see Gelb

1998). The government has argued that it remains committed to the aims of the RDP (and presumably to its housing agenda), and that GEAR provides a macroeconomic framework within which the objectives of the RDP can be met. These claims are somewhat belied by the fact that the chair of the RDP post was demoted from a cabinet-level position at the same time as GEAR was introduced. In other words and at best, instead of the aims of the RDP informing government policy, economic policy now seems to inform the RDP.

The GEAR document was developed and written for the Department of Finance by a technical team of economists. Almost all were white and male. Also, two were World Bank economists, and given that women have not fared particularly well under the directives of World Bank officials elsewhere in Africa and beyond, we might assume that the proposed cutbacks in public spending will affect South African women more severely than men (for examples of the dire and gendered effects of cutbacks in public spending in other African contexts and not least of all in aiding the spread of HIV, see Kirmani and Munyakho 1996). None of the models informing GEAR take particular account of the role of women in South Africa as either producers or consumers. In fact, the GEAR strategy as a whole does not adopt any gender perspectives on economic policy (Valodia 1998). According to GEAR, growth of the South African economy will be achieved through three primary growth drivers: exports, private investment, and change in the employment-growth relationship. The last of these, the employment-growth relationship, is meant to bring about a more labor-absorptive pattern of growth than has been the case to date: South Africa lost 4 percent of its formal-sector jobs between 1997 and 1998 (SAIRR 1998). Based on the fact that housing will become a localized governmental issue with national support,[2] and added to that shift in responsibility the fact that the economic empowerment of women does not shape national policy, the outlook for women as consumers of housing is pretty bleak.

Gendering Hostel Alternatives

At the local municipal level, hostel-upgrading schemes require a consensus of hostel opinion. It is therefore important to understand the social texture of hostels before consensus-building initiatives are set in place. To bring about the effective inclusion of hostel dwellers in the hostel-upgrading schemes, the organizing framework that governs hostel life must inform these policy decisions. It is at this level, perhaps, that the disempowering effect of heteropatriarchal planning is most evident.

As evidence, all the women living in the KwaThema hostel and interviewed for this project were reluctant to participate in the hostel's organizational structures. Interviews undertaken over three years found that women living in hostels did not participate in discussions about upgradings. Their isolation from the process was seen as a result not of their identity as women in the hostel, but rather of their impermanence—which is tied more to their historical status as women under apartheid and a problem of representation at the national level. Playing the role that ensures her survival, that of female migrant, the respondent, who had lived in the hostel for five years, distances herself from the upgradings underway: "I am not involved with the politics here. I am aware of the upgradings but *I am not permanent,* so it is not my place to talk or participate in these discussions. I cannot say what I want from authorities, or expect to have any say in how the hostel is run."[3] Another woman, who had been there two years, explained her distancing from the upgrading thus: "I am aware of the upgradings, but have only heard about it through hearsay. I have never actually seen evidence of it taking place."[4] Added to that, a spin-off of the upgrade for hostel residents is that they faced, on average, a 300 percent rent increase (Cullinan 1993a), a hike few could afford. In fact, the widely held perception that the hostel upgradings will lead to an increase in rent makes many hostel dwellers, especially those who are women, reticent about the planned upgrading: "I am not concerned about the upgradings; it is not for me to say. The hostel is a roof for me. . . . I can afford it. At this point I am grateful for that. I am worried that when the conversion happens, I will have to move anyway . . . so why bother with it now?"[5]

During a pilot upgrading scheme in a township neighboring Kwa-Thema, only 1.4 percent of the male hostel population were found to be satisfied with the upgradings that had taken place (Cullinan 1993b). This low measure of success is at first surprising, because the upgrading initiatives included an improvement in the storm water drainage system, the installation of hot water tanks and electrical outlets, and the repair of all broken windows. A follow-up report showed that the dissatisfaction stemmed from even male hostel dwellers' feelings of alienation from the upgrading process, and the fact that new measures had not included provisions for bedroom privacy.

This dissatisfaction demonstrates that the physical plans to upgrade hostels, although important, should also take the personal and historical consequences of apartheid planning into account (see fig. 7.1). As part of that process, the denial of privacy was one characteristic of apartheid; another was the subtle way in which women were discriminated against.

Deeply entrenched in the hostel-upgrading initiatives, and as a consequence of women's marginalization from the planning process, is a heteropatriarchal model of housing that serves to prolong the oppressive structures that women in hostel families have sought to resist and overcome. Evident in the upgrading plans is a reinscription of heterosexual male-headed families wherein "father knows best" or, at best, families visit for short periods. This familial ideal inscribed in space erases a history of resistance as well as viable and prudent housing initiatives developed by families in the cracks of the crumbling apartheid system. Missing from the current plans to upgrade hostels are the collective spaces for child care organized by women. Missing too are the attempts to blur public and private spaces. These planned spaces are designed solely as private spaces and so they undercut any attempts whereby families can gainfully work in the informal sector from their homes.

Turning toward that point as a possible avenue for future research, how should we begin to think about the new South African city? The architectural transformations put forward by planners to date manifest the heterospatialities of apartheid. The "family housing option" is a spatial design that emerges out of a highly contested debate on both the national and local scales. Implicit in that debate has been the continual marginalization of hostel dwellers' input and, in particular, voices of women who live in hostels. While the results from interviews for this study suggest that most women were not interested in participating in the formal discussions about the form that future housing took, the informal, yet visible, efforts that women living in the KwaThema hostel took to rebuild and reshape their environment suggest that alternative structures for negotiating the future must be sought.

Fig. 7.1. Original and upgrading hostel plans. One of the newer plans reveals a spatial reinscription of the heteropatriarchal family: a parental "master" bedroom with a double bed and a second bedroom with single beds for children.

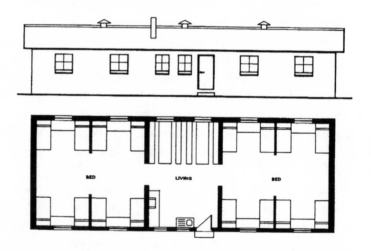

Existing hostel unit. Five interleading rooms, the central one of which allows access to the unit and contains two concrete dining tables with benches and a kitchen area with a sink and a coal stove. Public washroom and toilet facilities are located away from sleeping quarters.

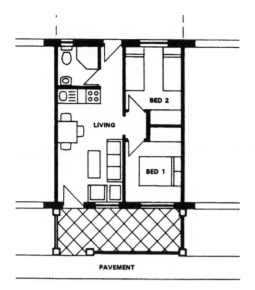

A second upgrading plan, this one a self-contained two-bedroom unit. This type (and its derivatives) is designed as a starter family unit for ownership or rental and can be upgraded to a two-story unit.

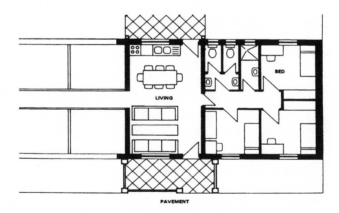

Example of an upgrading plan, featuring single rooms with access to shared ablutions, kitchen, and living area. This type (and its derivatives) is designed for communal living, or for either individual-title or rentable single-room accommodation—for those who are in a slightly higher income bracket but need to retain a rural home (or for residents who do not wish to relocate their families). This plan allows for overnight guests.

Women living in hostels have shown that they have skills to create a viable local economy there, premised on innovative uses of hostel space that include agriculture, retail activity, and animal husbandry, for example. In an attempt to rethink how these efforts could be integrated into future planning and having documented the debate leading to these plans, we now turn to a feminist agenda for direction.

Prospects for Future Research: Women, Housing Design, and Structure

Women who live in the hostels doubly feel the marginalization the hostel experienced at the national and local scale. The experience of these women and a gendered history of hostels prompt a number of questions concerning the future upgrading program. For example, how will gender relations be configured in hostel spaces as they are transformed into family housing? In what way will the gendered past of apartheid influence present family housing plans? How will the gendered spatial politics of apartheid and housing manifest themselves in these transformed buildings?

Conceptualizing housing space from a gendered perspective requires that we move beyond the physicality of the building and its form and focus instead on the architectural form as an embodiment of gendered social and physical spatial relations. Henri Lefebvre's observation reveals how traditional conceptualizations of housing have failed to move beyond the materiality of housing design: "In the light of an imaginary analysis, our house would emerge as permeated from every direction by streams of energy which run in and out of it by every imaginable route: water, gas, electricity, telephone lines, radio and television signals and so on. Its image of immobility would then be replaced by an image of a complex of mobilities, a nexus of in and out conduits" (1991, 93). Lefebvre's imaginary analysis of the house is useful in assisting gender-blind hostel planners to view the hostel as more than a physical construct, a discrete space. Present upgrading schemes propose to reshape the apartheid landscape simply by connecting the migrant worker hostels to electricity and water. Taking our cue from the analysis laid out here and recalling Grosz's (1995) reminder that housing is about sex, we turn our attention to the upgrading of hostel space specifically.

Although physical upgradings are important, the changing material conditions of daily life in hostels at present must also be related to a social urban history. Those connections include links to an apartheid past that represented hostels and hostel dwellers as marginal, disempowered, and heteromasculine. The conversion of hostel spaces must address the identity that has been constructed around them and the identity of hostel residents. Doing that requires that hostels be reintegrated into the township community. Innovative town-planning measures that create township foot traffic through the hostel, such as those proposed by Rubenstein (1993), are an example.[6] Beyond manipulating the physical landscape, however, it is important to overcome the organizational obstacles that stand in the way of adequate and fair housing provision. To date, this has not occurred.

The resulting architectural proposals that emerged from the five-year debate about hostel reform in KwaThema suggest that black women are not primary consumers of housing. Presently, women gain access to housing only as members of a family. Furthermore, the proposed designs fail to recognize the increasing numbers of single women who are currently housed in hostels.

South Africa is, of course, not unique in its disregard for women's housing. Within the context of U.S. public housing programs, an emerging feminist critique has taken shape. Among several broad-ranging issues raised by feminists is how the heterosexual, nuclear, male-headed family model is reinforced historically and in current public housing (see Nast and Wilson 1994). Debates from other settings reveal the consequence of ignoring the role of women in housing. Most recently, feminist architect Lisa Weisman has argued, "The housing problem that many people are experiencing results from ubiquitous sexism, racism, and classism that characterize patriarchal society. Housing, like affirmative action, reproductive freedom, or equal pay belongs on the feminist agenda" (1994, 115). Through an examination of the "man-made" environment, Weisman argues that "a woman's sexuality is defined by her spatial location"; that the "virtuous" woman is found in the nuclear-family house, the "whore" in the house of ill repute and in the embodiment of any woman who dares to walk the street at night (3). A similar assumption has informed the debate on the architecture of hostels, which have left no room for women as independent working individuals. The designs still create a false binary between those who are linked to a husband and are housed and those who do not have a "male-based" right to housing.

The "placement" of women in an apartheid history, their position in relation to hostels (see chapter 5), and existing power structures must inform upgrading schemes. The kinds of demands that women have as housing consumers were hinted at throughout many of the interviews conducted for this project. Although many women were silent when asked about the hostels directly, we gleaned extensive information from extended conversations. One four-year female resident noted the following: "I am only a visitor here; it is not my place to make any kind of judgment. One of the benefits of being here is the cheap rent. I would expect that to change. Although the conditions are bad at the moment, it still makes my life easier."[7] The statement reflects a history of marginalization and impermanence, a need for affordable housing and a fear of future displacement because of anticipated increases in rents when conversion takes place. Another respondent, who had lived in the KwaThema hostel for three years, argued, "When the conversions come through, I will have to move. The cheaper accommodation which is offered by hostels at present will change—at the moment I can provide for my children and operate a beer business—at R75 per month [the proposed rent amount] this will not be possible."[8] Beyond the immediate call for affordable housing, the quote also demonstrates that the contemporary South African landscape is already informed by a set of assumptions that distance many from direct involvement. Political sidelining and insufficient formal economic resources generated by women, who lived in KwaThema's hostel when this research was conducted, will result in their permanent displacement.

Making sense of the apartheid landscape continues to shape contemporary thinking and remains an important challenge for planners and policymakers in contemporary South Africa. One way to theorize the structures of inequality that shape spatial relations in South Africa involves the careful detailing of how decision makers wield power and how that power finally results in physical forms. That task extends beyond the physical spatial relations of architecture toward a spatial analysis that embraces a sensitivity to the way in which spatial meaning is constructed in social terms.

Once the web of power that shapes the landscape is understood, we also begin to note that the bulk of power lies in the hands of male urban actors. The apartheid landscape is not just any landscape but one that operated as a map upon which the procreational economy of apartheid operated. In fact, that procreational geography of apartheid continues. The landscape is one on which the power imbalance is particularly significant for women who live in South Africa's cities. For them, the transfer of power from a white minority to a black majority does not circumvent the particular heterosexism that informed apartheid. Empowering women marginalized by apartheid is as important to contemporary South Africa as understanding its racial imbalances. Indeed, empowering women may hold the key to reversing racial inequality. Nobel economics laureate Amartya Sen, informed by the South Asian context, has put it thus: "The changing agency of women is one of the major mediators of economic and social change, and its determination as well as consequences closely related to many of the central features of the development process" (1999, 202). The active participation of women as agents of change in South Africa, however, requires an epistemological space to be created wherein women as subjects are recognized and heard. As Grosz (1995) points out, this is clear: unless men can invent other ways to occupy space, unless space (territorialized, as mappable or explorable) gives way to place (occupation, dwelling, and being lived in), until space is conceived in terms other than according to the logic of penetration, colonization, and domination, unless men understand the necessity of according women their own space and negotiate the occupation of shared spaces, unless they no longer regard space as the provenance of their own expression and self-creation, unless they respect spaces and places that are not theirs, entering only when invited and accepting the invitation as a gift, men cannot share in the contributions that women may have to offer in reconceiving space and place.

The lived experiences of women in the cracks of apartheid are visions of resistance and survival. Collective strategies by women to raise families through national networks, create income in the informal economy, and miraculously survive in hostels must inform the low-cost housing programs in South Africa if an emancipatory city is to be fully realized.

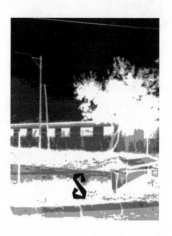

CHANGING THE SUBJECT

THE INTENTION of this study has been to lay out in time and space the manifold and complicated ways in which a process of impoverishment and marginalization has occurred. A further aim of the study has been to document the powerful ways in which many South Africans, but women in particular, lived on and resisted the procreational geography of apartheid. The conclusions and implications of this study are laid out within the pressing context of a health crisis. In other words, how and why do the procreational assumptions of apartheid, laid out in the geography of apartheid, continue to haunt South Africa's most impoverished people today?

Economic and political marginalization, social isolation, dislocation, stereotyping, sexual and political violence, and gender inequities are some of the social conditions that people living in hostels have endured. Unfortunately, those conditions are not dissimilar to the social circumstances under which South African people living with HIV and AIDS in contemporary South Africa seek survival. In other words, unchecked cycles of marginalization will continue to haunt South Africa until the challenges of the procreational economy of apartheid are confronted. One way of doing that is by altering the material legacy of the procreational economy etched on the landscape.

The resistant actions by women documented in these pages also serve as practical solutions. Acts of resistance can be seen as such when set against a complicated heteropatriarchal system configured in time and space. Explaining part of that strategy, one woman hostel resident explained: "There are three of us who have worked here, in the KwaThema hostel, since 1985. Children, permits, illnesses and deaths in Msinga, harvesting. We are never here together. The three of us make it possible for us to keep our hand in the hostel beer market and look after affairs at home. We also avoid the police if we are not living in the hostel for long periods. It's easier for women to avoid notice if they keep moving."[1]

By recontextualizing the lives of those interviewed for this study within historical time and geographical space, we see the pernicious and hitherto undocumented procreational geography of apartheid. A widowed mother of three put it so: "What choices do I have? I must move to survive. I must cut my body in two. My children live in Msinga now, but work and income is here. . . . To stand still is to die."[2] What follows here then is not only a synopsis of the argument laid out in this study, but also a treatise to action.

The Road Forward

The South African constitution that passed into law in 1996 states: "The state may not unfairly discriminate directly or indirectly against anyone on one or more grounds, including race, *gender, sex, pregnancy, marital status,* ethnic or social origin, colour, *sexual orientation,* age, disability, religion, conscience, belief, culture, language and birth" (South Africa 1996, 7; emphasis mine). This constitution, without doubt, marks a stunning break with the apartheid past and is worthy of the international praise it received, particularly in view of the bold, unprecedented step undertaken by this fledgling democracy to protect sexual orientation. However, examining the new constitution also reveals that of the seventeen protected identities listed, five (gender, sex, pregnancy, martial status, and sexual orientation) are elements that relate to redressing the effects of the procreational economy of apartheid. In other words, by making explicit mention of gender, sex, pregnancy, martial status, and sexual orientation, constitutional framers sought to undermine the consummate historical claims to heteropatriarchal power that some men through time and space have made in South Africa. Moreover, the new constitution seeks to provide a legal point from which to resist the historical, rhetorical, economic, and spatial implications of apartheid.

As surprising as the list of protected identities seems at first, we note through this study that these various elements have historically been part of the apartheid order. Identities, beyond racial proscriptions, were always intertwined in mutually reinforcing ways to ensure the smooth operation of apartheid. A reversal of apartheid discrimination requires a nonstatic understanding of identity more broadly, not simply a reversal of racism. One way of doing that is by reimagining gender and sexual identity outside the conventional heteronormative tropes that accord with the dictates of the apartheid procreational economy and are reflected in its heterospatiality or geography. By unpacking the spatial material legacy of apartheid and seeking the contours of the procreational economy within that spatial legacy, viable alternative strategies become imaginable. Put another way, redressing the inequalities of apartheid laid out in space, and doing so from a sexual perspective, is an efficient and timely strategy that provides an avenue for reimagining a just and equitable future for South Africa's most needy.

The task that now faces the new government is to put this theory into practice. We have noted that negotiating just change in South Africa is an inherently geographical exercise infused with the politics of sexuality. Said (1993) reminds us, in the opening to *Culture and Imperialism,* that decolonization processes are about transformation in the meaning of spaces. If we choose to interrogate the geography of apartheid or the meaning of its spatial legacy, we come to see that apartheid was in fact not simply a racial order but also one that was underpinned by a procreational economy. In other words, what held the system in place along with brutality, intended impoverishment, and dependence was an assumed heteronormative desire that could be strung out across space and time.

However, what translated into a spatial system with built-in assumptions about the value of men's mobility and women's immobility also became the spatial matrix within which women in particular challenged its boundaries. Sometimes those acts of defiance and resistance were literal spatial transgressions against gendered influx control laws. At other times, resistance against the imposed procreational economy of apartheid was a simple act of sending money to a loved one living in a hostel miles away. It might be argued that such gestures further exploited the black household in the interests of white capital. However, women who sent money, or lent support, understood their actions as necessary reversals of the vectors of designed and mapped heteropatriarchal dependence:

> Since '82 I've been coming to the hostel to visit my husband. In the beginning it was just for visits. After he lost his job in '84, I kept coming to visit, bringing him food, clothes. I stayed for three months and sold food here in the hostel to make money for us. In '87 he worked again but the money was not enough. In '88 he was killed. I now come back to make some money for our kids at home.[3]

To bring about a truly transformative politics requires that we make sense of the changing South African map by questioning specific spaces within the South African geographic imagination. To do that we can call into question the procreational assumptions that led to the location of spaces and places. To unpack the apartheid landscape we must assume that the static closed spaces of apartheid—the black township, the policed hostels, bureaucratic homelands—were static, herteronormatively imagined spatial inventions of an apartheid order. However, rather than closed, sealed spaces, their boundaries were and remain permeable. One way of subverting those static meanings is by recontextualizing them both spatially and historically within the politics of heterosexual desire. Instead of seeing the apartheid landscape as divided up and racialized, we can see spaces as interrelated and identities as interconnected through the politics of a constructed, racialized, heterosexed form of desire.

Employing this framework, we come to see not only how spaces relate to each other but also how identities in South Africa were tied to each other—or mutually constituted. For example, the identity *Zulu female* under apartheid is meaningless without understanding how that social signifier exists in counterdistinction to the idea of Zulu maleness. Under apartheid, the term *Zulu female*, once affixed, operated to the exclusion of all others. Indeed, a social identity locates its signified bearer in a grid of intelligibility (both social and spatial), determining, among other things, geographical mobility and access to power. In turn, these composite and complicated meanings become the building blocks of a racialized typology that developed into the social system called apartheid.

Results from this study show that when we examine the sexual dimensions of an apartheid space, like the hostel, that space comes to signify a multiplicity of purposes. While the hostel was an important component in the racial economy of South Africa (a point well documented in the literature), it is also a site of familial resistance, especially for women. We note too that hostels also operated as sites where family members (including women and children) resisted and co-opted the imposition of heteronormatized identities that would have otherwise destroyed their household and family structures. When the apartheid state launched its attack on the black family with influx control, thereby hoping to turn black family members into a heteronormatized and gendered (but differentially valued) workforce, the hostel was at the center of the struggle by most black working people to hold their families together. Speaking spatially, the reinscription of the heteropatriarchal differed from any former patriarchal regime because the procreational economy of apartheid created a procreational geography that extended over the national space of South Africa. By reinterpreting the meaning of hostel space, we see also that women continued to provide for their children and aging relatives from inside the hostel. In municipal hostels, men and women collectively supported each other and those in the rural reserves. By incorporating the hostel into the spatial network of survival, many families, if we imagine them outside heteronormative reasoning, were not destroyed.

For hostel dwellers today, the meaning of the hostel emerges as resultant vectors in geometry of survival and resistance strategies, apartheid and postapartheid oppression, and familial patriarchal domination. We see that the hostel as an apartheid state–engineered ideal was never realized because it was resisted, co-opted, and incorporated into an extended household structure by hostel dwellers who never passively accepted their racial prescriptions.

The linkages between areas of origin and the hostel are also at the core of the struggle for identity that hostel dwellers have experienced since the collapse of apartheid. The physical incarceration of hostel dwellers behind barbed-wire fences, and their symbolic imprisonment since the abolition of apartheid, secured by a discourse that labels their living spaces as fortresses of fear has isolated hostel dwellers' urban experience. Struggles over the meaning of hostels have marginalized hostel dwellers (women and children as well as men) in such a way that the path is left open to a stereotyping and postapartheid exploitation.

These debates reveal that for many South Africans not caught up in the migrant labor system during apartheid, the hostel was a terra incognita, and so in contemporary South Africa it is open to speculation and generalization. One way of breaking open the apartheid legacy is through a historically and spatially sensitive understanding of space and place. Furthermore, once we break open the fixedness of apartheid spaces by asking questions about the politics of desire and sex they represent, we also begin to see how apartheid as an order was constituted by a series of identities that went way beyond a simple racial classification.

Rather, apartheid was and remains a system that relied on the manipulation of sexual and therefore gendered relations, the regulation of sexuality through a gamut of laws that prohibited sex across color lines, between same-sex partners, and so on. Part of the challenge of the contemporary moment is to unravel the combined way in which identity was used in South Africa. Context-specific homophobia, sexism, and ethnic discrimination in fact were all necessary parts of an apartheid order, processes that were manipulated to support the *myth* of race. Translating that theoretical notion into real politics involved the slow and careful unpacking of the interconnected spatial relations that define the contemporary landscape. That unpacking of spatial relations translates into examining how inherently spatial processes, like migration, are understood by those who participate in them.

Translating Theory into Practice

Policy Implications of the Study

While the hostel is a site that resonates in current urban theoretical debates, it is also a site of topical significance for urban policymakers in South Africa: "While hostels are manifestly inadequate institutions, they both contain and have created certain social realities that will not go away with the dismantling of the physical structure" (*Star*, 8/28/95). This statement by Lawrence Schlemmer, one of South Africa's foremost policy analysts, that South Africa's hostels have both physical and social dimensions, received widespread criticism (*Star*, 8/29/95; *Citizen*, 8/29/95; *Sowetan*, 8/30/95). The press and the ensuing public policy debate, quite incorrectly, interpreted his statements as an argument for retaining the hostel system.

Criticism of Schlemmer's statement provides hints about popularly held policy perceptions in South Africa. A more accurate reading of his statement would have shown that in fact he was arguing that a dismantling of the hostels would not end the social reality of apartheid; apartheid was more than the built environment and its legacy is more than its constituent parts. Urban public policy debates must move forward and take that position.

Institutional Transformation

Policy directions must not address apartheid simply as a racial order. The results of this research have shown that local political institutions—like municipalities, city councils, and civic organizations—while effective in resisting the racial injustices of apartheid, are not the most efficient structures within which to negotiate the future. Antiracist institutions will not effectively redress the apartheid past. As institutions they were forged in the resistance politics of apartheid and, while local organizations engaged in heroic struggles against the larger apartheid social structure, they were not democratic institutions. The subversive, highly censored, and dangerous political environment of black townships during the 1980s created a political elite who organized locally and with a high level of independence and limited accountability.

The scramble for power and legitimacy during the late 1980s as apartheid crumbled and during the multiparty elections in 1994 has left several antiapartheid institutions, like civic committees and hostel dweller committees, warped by party politics. Unfortunately, as existing institutional structures, these organizations have thus far provided the framework within which most transformative policies have operated. This study has demonstrated that the creation of more inclusive, long-term organizational structures should also be built into future policy initiatives. To bring about that kind of postapartheid political restructuring, attention must be paid to the way in which apartheid also oppressed individuals in their capacity as workers, members of ethnic or religious minorities, sexual beings, senior citizens and children, and language speakers if the precepts of the new constitution are going to be upheld by the Constitutional Court. These differences, and the way in which they are linked to racism, must be explored more fully and reflected in the institutional political organization.

Nation building cannot occur along racial lines, especially if the category of race remains unproblematized. A nuanced analysis of identity more broadly must inform those efforts.

To demonstrate the danger of a static understanding of race and how it continues to flourish in contemporary South Africa, I quote at length from the statements of President Thabo Mbeki:

> A major component part of the issue of reconciliation and nation-building is defined by and derives from the material conditions in our society which have divided our country into two nations, the one black and the other white.
>
> We therefore make bold to say that South Africa is a country of two nations.
>
> One of these nations is white, relatively prosperous, regardless of gender or geographical dispersal. It has ready access to a developed economic, physical, educational, communication and other infrastructure. This enables it to argue that, except for persistence of gender discrimination against women, all members of this nation have the possibility to exercise their right to equal opportunity, the development opportunities to which the Constitution of 1993 committed our country.
>
> The second, larger nation in South Africa is black and poor, with the worst affected being women in the rural areas, the black rural population, and the disabled. This nation lives under conditions of a grossly underdeveloped economic, physical, educational, communication and other infrastructure. It has virtually no possibility to exercise what in realty amounts to a theoretical right to equal opportunity, with that right being equal within this black nation only to the extent that it is equally incapable of realisation.

This reality of two nations, underwritten by the perpetuation of the *racial, gender* and *spatial disparities* born of a very long period of colonial and apartheid white minority domination, constitutes the material base which reinforced the notion that, indeed, we are not one nation, but two nations. (1998, 72, my emphasis)

I have not quoted the present president to discount the material inequality that he accurately observes. In fact, the conditions described above serve to reinforce the dire levels of rural poverty described in this study. Rather the purpose of quoting Mbeki at length lies in my concern with the fixed way in which dichotomies of race operate in his narrative. According to Mbeki, the inequalities of gender and geography are quirks of race, not constituent parts. In his description of the state of the South African nation, we see two worlds: one white, one black. The gender inequalities experienced by white South African women, while mentioned, are glossed over by the president while the experiences of Indian and Coloured South Africans are ignored altogether. It is not a coincidence that, by the president's own admission, "the worst affected [are black] women in rural areas." Missed by the president is how gender and sexual inequality are the very building blocks of race in South Africa. Race as configured under apartheid was an endpoint. That dichotomy cannot mark the starting point for unpacking apartheid's effect. The gross rendering of the South African condition by the sitting president is troubling.

Conceptual Transformations

As this study has shown, in the case of the hostel transformation projects, negotiators have ignored the politics of heterosexuality that shape hostels and the lives of increasing numbers of women living in hostels. Not only is this oversight unfair, it also overlooks many of the cost-effective and informal measures that individuals have negotiated in the cracks of apartheid.

The hostel where this research was conducted presents an interesting theoretical challenge to our thinking but also a challenge to conventional urban planning. Traditional dichotomies like urban and rural, work and home, industrial and residential are blended and reworked in the survival strategies of hostel dwellers. Accordingly, these sites, which were deregulated during South Africa's transformation, are also fertile sites for exploring the ingenious and inventive survival strategies of families, particularly the strategies employed by women living in hostels.

Bearing in mind the limited financial resources of local authorities, other nonmaterial resources, like an "economy of affection," must find value within this context. Indeed, a recent study in KwaZulu-Natal concluded, "In the light of . . . problems that are engendered by IMF-style development . . . analysis of group and individual interactions can lead to a more sensitive understanding of how social factors through the economy of affection, give way to more creative thinking about ways in which to empower self-employed women" (Singh 1999, 485). Economies of affection stand in stark contrast to the procreational economy of apartheid. The malevolent geographies of apartheid sought to create heteropatriarchal architectures of patronage, assistance, and desire. By contrast, the economy of affection is a nonhierarchical communal system of support. Within these more benevolent geographies are found the resistant survival strategies that extend over space and have developed within the cracks of apartheid's heterospatiality. Outside of the spatiality of the argument, this view, of course, is not revolutionary or new. Amartya Sen's *Development as Freedom,* puts is thus: "Nothing, arguably, is as important today in the political economy of development as an adequate recognition of the political, economic and social participation and leadership of women. This is indeed a crucial aspect of 'development as freedom'" (1999, 203). In spaces like collapsing hostel buildings we find examples: collective childcare arrangements and sequential migration arrangements among women who move back and forth between home and Msinga. These are two strategies used by women who have negotiated limited budgets in order to survive. These are valuable visions for future policymakers.

Regional and local planning initiatives must work in collaborative projects that subvert the procreational geography of apartheid. Migration to the KwaThema hostel will continue until women are physically barred (which would be a return to old-style apartheid), or until adequate social welfare agencies that provide education and economic opportunities are put in place in Msinga. Similarly, the hostel community will not be incorporated in township life until the physical and emotional fences are removed through creative town-planning projects.

Turning to the hostel conversions specifically, we see that women's survival networks provide planners with a map of the flows of support that need to be incorporated into future family housing and not simply erased to be replaced with "family housing." Stepping outside heteronormatized patterns and choosing to live in hostels, acting as care providers and earning income, women have negotiated their survival. Future hostel plans should actively encourage the establishment of informal and formal retail activities. Along with providing space for these activities, short-term, low-interest loans or credit for collective business ventures by hostel dwellers would be one way to build on the existing informal economy. Several upgrading efforts have proposed that unemployed hostel dwellers receive on-the-job training as builders during the upgrading process. These innovative strategies must advance, however, beyond the concept that all hostel dwellers are men. Women are and always have been connected to the hostels and must therefore be involved in their transformation.

Creating a context within which these strategies are recognized is difficult. The strategies that women have adopted are all but invisible, and the challenge lies in creating institutions that would promote visibility for the strategies and desires of marginalized groups.

These suggestions also have serious limitations and we should not romanticize their significance. Rather, what we can conclude is that unraveling the complex, contradictory nature, as well as the inefficiencies, of apartheid is an important task for the present. Part of that effort involves moving away from the static "truths" of apartheid (like racial identity and bounded spaces) and allowing policy to be shaped by the ways in which working people under apartheid and under present-day circumstances survive. Part of that effort must also involve creating an epistemological space where the subjectivities of women, in particular, are acknowledged.

To unlock these strategies requires alternative research strategies. In an attempt to rethink ways of unlocking these processes, this study sought to document life in a fluid and rapidly changing contemporary South Africa through a qualitative research procedure. It is to the direction of future research that we now turn.

Mapping the New Spaces

Through this study we note the way in which the imposed heterosexual-ized politics of apartheid continue to inform the geographical imaginings of contemporary South Africans. The hostel is a particularly fascinating context and metaphor for exploring the connection between the procre-ational economy of the apartheid landscape and its undetected effects on the future. We have seen that the hostel held significance for all South Africans, not only those who lived its material reality. At the level of rep-resentation, for example, the hostel held meaning for the construction of whiteness and blackness, maleness and femaleness. The politics of daily life are not solely grounded in the material world. Evidence presented here suggests that daily life for black South African men and women is more complicated than a struggle against racism. Daily life and the ne-gotiation of a heterosexualized identity (which includes but is not limited to racial proscription) is one of the sites where the politics of the mate-rial and representational spheres intersect. Daily life is a negotiation of both elements and takes place in and through space. The evidence sug-gests that while the politics of transformation in South Africa must ad-dress material politics, that focus cannot adequately redress the material and representational legacy of apartheid.

The hostel is also a metaphor for unpacking the material and repre-sentational politics of space. Hostel space also lends itself to investigating the construction and meaning of other apartheid spaces: for our purposes the hostel serves a particular function as a heterosexualized space.

We see throughout the study that the geographic mode of analysis is a particularly powerful tool with which to assist in the transformation of South Africa and that an important part of South Africa's transition to democracy is a geographic exercise.

Implications for a Contemporary HIV Policy in South Africa

In light of these findings, critics might charge that any compelling case for studying the procreational geography of apartheid has been supplanted by the pressing demands of HIV in South Africa. However, deeply trou-bling HIV statistics should also be placed in the broader contours of the procreational geography of apartheid. Indeed, the politics of HIV transmission between men and women and vice versa must be understood from a gender-sex perspective. Once we grasp that the differential claims to power of men and women—and in particular migrant men and women—exist because of the still-present procreational geography of apartheid, we can begin to imagine proactive strategies that will stem the tide of HIV transmission in South Africa. The following newspaper account graphically highlights those challenges and echoes many of the themes of gender-sex violence examined earlier:

NEIGHBORS KILL AN HIV-POSITIVE AIDS ACTIVIST IN SOUTH AFRICA

A volunteer working to persuade South Africans not to discriminate against HIV-infected people was beaten to death last week by her neighbors, who accused her of bringing shame on their community by revealing that she was HIV-positive.

The killing scared other anti-AIDS advocates and said it proved what they have said for years—although 3 million South Africans are infected with the virus that causes AIDS, nearly all are afraid to admit it because of the hostility they face.

The woman killed, Gugu Dlamini, 36, a volunteer field worker for the National Association of People Living with HIV/AIDS, went public on World AIDS Day, Dec. 1, speaking about her HIV infection on Zulu-language radio and on television.

Since then, according to nurses who knew her, she was repeatedly threatened by neighbors in her township of KwaMashu, outside Durban, who said she was giving their community a bad reputation.

Last Monday, she was punched and slapped by a man who told her that many others who were sick kept quiet about it.

South Africa has the world's fastest-growing AIDS epidemic, according the latest UNAIDS reports, and KwaZulu-Natal, where Ms. Dlamini lived, is the worst-hit province. Up to 30 percent of adults there are infected. Although Ms. Dlamini called the police that day, they did nothing, friends told a local newspaper. That night, a mob attacked her house and stoned her, kicked her and beat her with sticks. She died the next day.

"She was a nice, bright woman, and now her child is an orphan because of AIDS," said Mercy Makhalemele, a Durban-area administrator for the association.

"But not because she died of it. Because she was trying to exercise her constitutional right to freedom of speech."

A spokesman for the KwaZulu-Natal health department called the attack "sheer stupidity" and Deputy President Thabo Mbeki, who promoted AIDS awareness in his Christmas message to the nation, said: "It is a terrible story. We have to treat people who have HIV with care and support, and not as if they have an illness that is evil. (*New York Times*, December 28, 1998)

Four suspects were charged with Dlamini's murder but were released because, eyewitness accounts notwithstanding, there was not enough evidence to prosecute them (*Star,* 1/11/01).

How do we make sense of this murder? Perhaps Gugu Dlamini's killing should be contextualized within broader structures of public and domestic violence that has wracked South Africa for almost fifteen years. Perhaps her killing could be explained as the result of her having spoken when she should have observed the code of silence. Whatever conclusions we choose to draw, her killing was neither stupid nor inexplicable. To call this action "sheer stupidity" is an inappropriate response that hides the complex systems of oppression that continue to challenge the survival of women like Gugu Dlamini in contemporary South Africa.

Explaining elements of Gugu Dlamini's death and guaranteeing the survival of millions of women like her (like those interviewed for this study) could begin by way of an interrogation of the procreational economy of apartheid and its attendant landscape. Gugu Dlamini's killing outside a shebeen in KwaManchinza, an informal settlement near KwaMashu in KwaZulu Natal, also underscores that it is women living in KwaZulu Natal whom HIV has infected most savagely. Recall that a history of migrant labor has cut deeply into the social geography of this eroded landscape. A recent South African Medical Research Council report (Karim and Karim 1999) notes that the HIV prevalence rate (26.9 percent) is highest in KwaZulu Natal. Tying these figures to what we have come to understand in this study as the procreational economy of apartheid, the research council's study notes, "While the factors underpinning this gradient of infection have not been elucidated, urban-rural differences and differences in the levels of migration partially account for this gradient"

(2). For many of the reasons laid out in this study, it is no coincidence that these women (like many interviewed for this study) are also South Africa's most HIV infected population. They are also the most socially, economically, and geographically disempowered.

The topic of HIV/AIDS at the conclusion of this study underscores the urgent need to address the topic in the midst of imagining social transformation. Also, understanding the spread of HIV in time and space, or its epidemiology in South Africa, might be informed by the geographical theory developed here. Many of the women interviewed for this study are also embroiled in the bloody and life-threatening patterns of heteropatriarchal violence, and a gendered analyses of violence must take center stage in deliberation about HIV in South Africa.

Lori Heise (1997) has argued that the failure of the global health community to recognize the gender-based abuse in light of the HIV crisis has put both important public health objectives and individual women at risk. She argues that by ignoring the pervasive violence within relationships, the current global AIDS strategy (which is based heavily on condom promotion) dooms itself to failure. A review of 2,100 articles from five of the top family-planning and health journals reveals that between 1980 and 1992, sexuality and male-female power dynamics are mentioned only within three narrow contexts: how women's attitudes about sexuality influence contraceptive use and effectiveness (41 articles); how adolescent attitudes about sexuality influence contraceptive use and are related to teen pregnancy (24 articles); and how "high risk" sexual behaviors are related to the spread of sexually transmitted diseases, including AIDS (11 articles) (Dixon-Mueller 1992).

What this research shows is why women are afraid to even broach the subject of condom use for fear of male reprisal. This is confirmed by other studies in other contexts (Elias and Heise 1993; Rao Gupta 1993). This disempowerment is worsened when we consider that many of the women interviewed for this study risk physical abuse but also the loss of shelter and housing. Even more alarming is that current efforts to upgrade old apartheid-style hostels into family housing have not taken the rising HIV rates into consideration. The heteronormatized politics of daily life in hostels created a climate in which women believe they stand to gain if they become pregnant. Even though this failed to be true in most cases, and most women living in the hostel in KwaThema were single mothers, the promise of male support and patronage is all too compelling for many of the women interviewed.

In 1997 the World Health Organization conservatively estimated that just under 3 million South Africans were infected with the virus that causes AIDS (approximately 12 percent of the adult population). These estimates, however, vary widely when particular sectors of South African society are examined in detail. Data suggests that 44 percent of young pregnant women in KwaZulu Natal are infected with HIV (*Mail and Guardian*, 5/7/99). At the time of writing, the South African government had turned down offers from Western nations to provide AZT to pregnant mothers, because, it was argued insufficient proof exists that such medications greatly minimize the transmission of the virus to children. The lack of infrastructure and financial resources to sustain such a program also helped the contemporary South African state to conclude it could not afford to "save" these women and children. Absent from the debate were the voices of young pregnant Zulu women. Just as drastic measures are needed to stem the tide of HIV, so too are imaginative and emancipatory ways of imagining and creating spaces in the cacophony that presently is the Rainbow Nation.

These figures unfortunately suggest that South Africa is one of the world's worst-affected countries. Given South Africa's attempt to move away from its apartheid past, the tragedy of HIV/AIDS is that it may achieve what the apartheid regime failed to do: remove black South Africans from the land of their birth. The effect of HIV/AIDS can be resisted if, and only if, heteropatriarchal attitudes and the spaces wherein those attitudes reside are rethought and rebuilt. The tokoloshe will be exorcised by policies that recognize black South African women as subjects who have inalienable rights that include organizing and imagining themselves outside procreational roles and geographies. Economies of affection established by women and in resistance to the procreational economy of apartheid are one example of how malevolent geographies are challenged and changed by more benevolent geographies. Providing women with empowering tools, like the more expensive female condoms instead of the cheaper male condoms, also requires a step away from heteropatri-archal attitudes and justifications that see women as expendable. Locating women along with men at the center of policy debates is one way of challenging the legacy of apartheid; it will also slow down the HIV/AIDS epidemic in South Africa.

ПOTES

Note: Field interviews were conducted at the KwaThema hostel between July 1993 and January 1994. Permission to interview hostel residents was gained from two different hostel committees and the hostel manager. Each female interviewee was assigned a Personal History Interview (PHI) number (1–30) to maintain confidentiality. The number after the PHI number denotes which interview is cited, so 16.2 is the second interview with respondent number sixteen. This number is followed by the date of the interview. Interviewees' names were not attached to interview schedules but maintained in a separate log.

Chapter 1

1. Personal History Interview 4.1, KwaThema hostel, September 28, 1993.
2. PHI 16.1, January 13, 1994.

Chapter 2

1. The Eastern Cape Province, comprising the former Ciskei and Transkei territories, extends along the southeastern coast of South Africa and also includes a small inland area encircled by KwaZulu-Natal.

2. "The toyi-toyi has developed into a show of strength," explains the ANC Department of Arts and Culture. "[I]t says we exist, we are here, you cannot easily forget about us!" (quoted in Reed 1994, 20). Apparently the *toyi-toyi* came to South Africa from the Zimbabwean guerrilla training camps, where it was used as a warm-up exercise by the Zimbabwean People's Revolutionary Army to boost fitness and morale. The toyi-toyi was, it seems, invented by the warriors of Mzilikazi, a renegade Zulu general who fled from the Zulu king Shaka, taking his regiments all the way to modern-day Zimbabwe. Legend has it that they started off from Zululand at a trot, hence the warlike, trotting rhythm of the toyi-toyi.

The dance came into vogue when ANC cadres (guerrilla officers), who were arrested while trying to infiltrate back into South Africa, taught it to their fellow detainees, who in turn spread it through the townships after their release. The toyi-toyi became the accepted norm at gatherings of the United Democratic Front, a broad alliance of antiapartheid organizations founded in Cape Town in 1983, which became the ANC's internal wing.

3. Informal discussion with woman informal trader outside the KwaThema hostel, August 22, 1993.

4. Interview with KwaThema hostel manager, July 7, 1993.

5. PHI 15.2, November 25, 1993.

6. For a detailed account of the regional tensions between the African National Congress government and the Inkatha Freedom Party in KwaZulu-Natal since the 1994 elections, see Alexander 1996.

Chapter 3

1. PHI 16.1, January 13, 1994.

2. At this point it is unclear whether the sex-gender system was put in place knowingly by planners, resulted from heteropatriarchal blindness on the part of authorities who devalued women's labor, reflected the fantasies and desires of rulers, or a combination thereof. In fact, the intent of the state lies outside the purview of this study, but certainly does provide a compelling set of questions for future research.

3. Another alternative for men was to buy goods and domestic services from newly arrived eastern European Jews (Sherman 2000; Elder 1997).

Chapter 4

1. PHI 18.1, November 1993.

2. PHI 17.1, January 14, 1994.

Chapter 5

1. Examples include Mayer 1961; Bundy 1972; Wilson 1972; Nelson 1976; Rosen-Prinz and Prinz 1978; R. Gordon 1977; E. Gordon 1981a, b; First 1983; Russell 1983, 1993; de Vletter 1985; Taylor 1990; Hanks and Lipire 1993. For a challenge to these accounts, see Sinclair 1998.

2. PHI 16.1, January 13, 1994.

3. PHI 16.2, January 20, 1994; emphasis mine.

4. Moodie asserts that "Bantu-speaking communities are not only patriarchal but also gerontocratic, organized on principles of seniority. Without respect for elders, the entire political and moral economy of traditional Bantu-speaking

societies would unravel" (1994, 129). This gerontocratic patriarchal organization was also reflected in the responses of Zulu-speaking women interviewed in this project. For example, the powerful social position of respondents' mothers-in-law was mentioned to me. Because most of the women interviewed had in fact fallen through the "traditional" rural networks, I would argue that the gerontocratic organizing principle of patriarchal relations was in fact relaxed. While old men were still held in high regard by the women interviewed, older women in the hostel did not hold any real influence over younger women. For this reason I have limited my analysis to the gendered dimensions of the patriarchal household system and for the purposes of this study will not examine the relationship between power and age.

5. For a superb account of the process of land expropriation, sharecropping, systematic impoverishment, and proletarianization throughout twentieth-century South Africa, see Van Onselen 1996.

6. PHI 5.1, September 28, 1993.

7. PHI 9.2, September 29, 1993.

8. PHI 16.2, January 20, 1994.

9. PHI 16.2, January 20, 1994.

10. PHI 22.2, January 22, 1994.

11. PHI 27.2, October 15, 1993.

12. Pseudonyms have been used to protect the identities of all respondents.

Chapter 7

1. This percentage was calculated from proposed expenditures in policy statements by the government before the budget figures were released (see, for example, Cobbett 1993) and from the total housing budget.

2. For details on hostels specifically, see Smit and Vedalankar 1993; for urban policy more generally, see Tomlinson 1994.

3. PHI 4.2, November 21, 1993; emphasis mine.

4. PHI 19.2, January 19, 1994.

5. PHI 20.2, January 22, 1994.

6. These examples include creating public footpaths through the hostel buildings. These public walkways serve to connect the hostel and the township.

7. PHI 18.2, January 19, 1994.

8. PHI 14.2, November 21, 1993.

Chapter 8

1. PHI 5.1, September 28, 1993.

2. PHI 11.1, October 2, 1993.

3. PHI 13.1, October 9, 1993.

BIBLIOGRAPHY

Newspapers Surveyed (1988–1994)

Argus, Cape Town.
Beeld, Johannesburg.
Burger, Die, Johannesburg.
Business Day, Johannesburg.
Cape Times, Cape Town.
Citizen, Johannesburg.
City Press, Johannesburg.
Daily Mail, Johannesburg.
Daily News, Johannesburg.
Diamond Fields Advertiser, Kimberley.
Evening Post, Kimberley.
Finance Week, Johannesburg.
Financial Mail, Johannesburg.
Finansies and Tegniek, Johannesburg.
Herald, Durban.
Kerkbode, Die, Pretoria.
Mayibuye, Durban.
Monitor, Cape Town.
Natal Mercury, Durban.
Natal Witness, Durban.
New Nation, Johannesburg.
Pretoria News, Pretoria.
Prisma, Johannesburg.

Rapport, Johannesburg.

Sowetan, Soweto.

Star, Johannesburg.

Sunday Star, Johannesburg.

Sunday Times, Johannesburg.

Sunday Tribune, Johannesburg.

Transvaler, Die, Johannesburg.

Volksblad, Die, Pretoria.

Vrye Weekblad, Pretoria.

Weekly Mail, Johannesburg.

Books and Articles

Achmat, Z. 1993. "'Apostles of Civilised Vice': 'Immoral Practices' and 'Unnatural Vice' in South African Prisons and Compounds, 1890–1920." *Social Dynamics* 19:92–110.

Adam, H., and K. Moodley. 1992. "Political Violence, 'Tribalism,' and Inkatha." *Journal of Modern African Studies* 30:485–510.

Adelzadeh, A. 1996. "From the RDP to GEAR: The Gradual Embracing of Neoliberalism in Economic Policy." *Transformation* 31:66–95.

Alexander, J. 1996. "Politics and Violence in KwaZulu-Natal." *Terrorism and Political Violence* 8:78–107.

Bazilli, S. 1991. *Putting Women on the Agenda.* Johannesburg: Ravan.

Beinart, W. 1987. "Worker Consciousness, Ethnic Particularism, and Nationalism." In *The Politics of Race, Class and Nationalism in Twentieth-Century South Africa,* ed. S. Marks and S. Trapido, 33–56. London: Longman.

Bond, P. 2000. *Cities of Gold, Townships of Coal: Essays on South Africa's New Urban Crisis.* Trenton, N.J.: Africa World Press.

Bond, P., and M. Khosa. 1999. *An RDP Policy Audit.* Pretoria: HSRC Publishers.

Bonner, P. 1990. "Desirable or Undesirable Women? Liquor, Prostitution, and the Migration of Basotho Women to the Rand, 1920–1945." In *Women and Gender in Southern Africa,* ed. C. Walker, 221–50. Cape Town: David Philip.

Bordo, S. 1999. *The Male Body: A New Look at Men in Public and Private.* New York: Farrar, Straus and Giroux.

Bozzoli, B. 1983. "Marxism, Feminism, and South African Studies." *Journal of Southern African Studies* 9 (2): 139–71.

———. 1985. "Migrant Women and South African Social Change: Biographical Approaches to Social Analysis." *African Studies* 44 (1): 87–96.

———— (with M. Nkotsoe). 1991. *Women of Phokeng: Consciousness, Life Strategy, and Migrancy in South Africa, 1900–1983.* Johannesburg: Ravan.

Brandel-Syrier, M. 1971. *Reeftown Elite: Social Mobility in a Black Community on the Johannesburg Reef.* New York: Africana Publishing Corporation.

Breckenridge, K. 1990. "Migrancy, Crime, and Faction Fighting: The Role of Isitshozi in the Development of Ethnic Organisations in Compounds." *Journal of Southern African Studies* 16 (1): 55–78.

Brink, B., R. Sher, and L. Clausen. 1986. *HIV Antibody Prevalence in South Africa during 1986.* South Africa: Chamber of Mines.

Brookes, E. 1991. "New Outlook on Mine Housing at Welkom." *Optima* 1:5–7.

Brown, B. 1983. "The Impact of Male Labour Migration on Women in Botswana." *African Affairs* 82:367–88.

Bundy, C. 1972. "The Emergence and Decline of the South African Peasantry." *African Affairs* 71:285–310.

Burawoy, M. 1972. "Another Look at the Mineworker." *African Social Research* 14:13–30.

Butler, J. 1990. *Gender Trouble: Feminism and the Subversion of Identity.* London: Routledge.

Campbell, C., G. Mare, and C. Walker. 1995. "Evidence for an Ethnic Identity in the Life Histories of Zulu-Speaking Durban Township Residents." *Journal of Southern African Studies* 21 (2): 287–301.

Carrier, J., and S. Murray. 1998. "Woman-Woman Marriage in Africa." In *Boy-Wives and Female Husbands: Studies of African Homosexualities,* ed. S. Murray and W. Roscoe, 255–66. New York: St. Martin's.

Chabram, A., and T. Fregoso. 1990. "Chicano/a Cultural Representations: Reframing Alternative Critical Discourses." *Cultural Studies* 4 (3): 201–16.

Chauhan, I. 1986. *The Dilemma of Working Women Hostelers: With Special Reference to Maharashtra.* New York: Stosius Inc., Advent Books Division.

Christopher, A. 1994. *The Atlas of Apartheid.* New York: Routledge.

Cobbett, W. 1993. "Redevelopment, ANC Style." *Reconstruct: A Work in Progress Supplement* 12:4.

Cock, J. 1980. *Maids and Madams: A Study in the Politics of Exploitation.* Johannesburg: Ravan.

————. 1989. *Maids and Madams: Domestic Workers under Apartheid.* 3d. ed. London: Women's Press.

Cohen, R. 1986. *Endgame in South Africa.* London: James Curry.

Cotterill, P. 1992. "Interviewing Women: Issues of Friendship, Vulnerability, and Power." *Women's Studies International Forum* 15:593–606.

Crush, J. 1991. "The Discourse of Progressive Human Geography." *Progress in Human Geography* 15 (4): 395–414.

———. 1992. "Power and Surveillance on the South African Gold Mines." *Journal of Southern African Studies* 18 (4), 825–43.

———. 1994. "Scripting the Compound." *Society and Space* 12 (3): 301–24.

Crush, J., and W. James. 1991. "Depopulating the Compounds: Migrant Labour and Mine Housing in South Africa." *World Development* 19:301–16.

Crush, J., A. Jeeves, and G. Yudelman. 1991. *South Africa's Labor Empire: A History of Black Migrancy to the Gold Mines.* Boulder: Westview.

Cullinan, K. 1993a. "No Success without Hostel Residents." *Reconstruct: A Work in Progress Supplement* 12:5.

———. 1993b. "NUM Tackles Living Conditions." *Reconstruct: A Work in Progress Supplement* 12:6–7.

de Kock, C., C. Schutte, N. Rhoodie, and D. Ehlers. 1993. "A Quantitative Analysis of Some Possible Explanations for the Hostel-Township Violence." In *Communities in Isolation: Perspectives on Hostels in South Africa.* Goldstone Hostels Report 1993, ed. A. Minnaar, 169–236. Pretoria: Human Sciences Research Council.

de Vletter, F. 1985. "Recent Trends and Prospects of Black Migration to South Africa." *Journal of Modern African Studies* 23 (4): 667–702.

Dixon-Mueller, R. 1992. *Sexuality, Gender, and Reproductive Health.* Working paper prepared for International Women's Health Coalition, New York.

Doran, J. 1990. *A Moving Issue for Women: Is Low Cost Transport an Appropriate Intervention to Alleviate Women's Burden in Southern Africa.* Norwich: University of East Anglia Press.

Dunstan, J. 1992. "Hostels: The Dilemma and the Challenge." *IPM Journal,* December–January.

Edwards, R. 1990. "Connecting Method and Epistemology: A White Woman Interviewing Black Women." *Women's Studies International Forum* 13 (5): 477–90.

Elder, G. 1990. "The Grey Dawn of South African Residential Integration." *GeoJournal* 22: 57–65.

———. 1997. "Decolonizing the 'Kaffir.'" *Jewish Affairs* 52 (3): 53–57.

———. 1998. "The South African Body Politic: Space, Race and Heterosexuality." In *Places through the Body,* ed. H. Nast and S. Pile, 153–64. London: Routledge.

Elias, C., and L. Heise. 1993. *The Development of Microbicides: A New Method of HIV Prevention for Women.* Programs Divisions Working Paper no. 6. New York: Population Council.

Fairhurst, J., I. Booysen, and P. Hattingh, eds. 1997. *Migration and Gender: Place,*

Time, and People Specific. Pretoria: University of Pretoria/International Geographical Union.

Finch, J. 1984. "'It's Great to Have Someone to Talk to': The Ethics and Politics of Interviewing Women." In *Social Researching: Politics, Problems, Practice,* ed. C. Bell and H. Roberts, 70–87. London: Routledge and Kegan Paul.

First, R. 1983. *Black Gold: The Mozambican Miner, Proletarian, and Peasant.* New York: St. Martin's Press.

Foucault, M. 1978. *The History of Sexuality.* Vol. 1, *An Introduction.* New York: Random House.

———. 1980. *Power/Knowledge: Selected Interviews and Other Writings, 1972-1977.* New York: Pantheon.

Freed, L. 1949. *The Problem of European Prostitution in Johannesburg: A Sociological Survey.* Johannesburg: Juta.

———. 1963. *Crime in South Africa: An Integralist Approach.* Johannesburg: Juta.

Friedman, M., and A. Wilkes. 1986. "Androcentric Knowledge and Geography—Examined?" *South African Geographical Journal* 65:89–94.

Furlong, P. 1994. "Improper Intimacy: Afrikaans Churches, the National Party, and the Anti-Miscegenation Laws." *South African Historical Journal* 31:55–79.

Gaitskell, D. 1979. "Christian Compounds for Girls: Church Hostels for African Women in Johannesburg, 1907–1970." *Journal of Southern African Studies* 6:44–69.

Gelb, S. 1998. "The Politics of Macroeconomic Reform in South Africa." Paper presented at the Conference on Democracy and the Political Economy of Reform, Cape Town.

Gevisser, M., and E. Cameron. 1995. *Defiant Desire: Gay and Lesbian Lives in South Africa.* New York: Routledge.

Gilroy, R., and R. Woods. 1994. *Housing Women.* London: Routledge.

Goodlad, R. 1996. "The Housing Challenge in South Africa." *Urban Studies* 33 (9): 1629–64.

Gordimer, N. 1953. *The Lying Days.* London: Victor Gollancz.

Gordon, D. 1991. "The Pafuri Camp." *Mining Survey* 2:32–41.

Gordon, E. 1981a. "Easing the Plight of Migrant Worker Families in Lesotho." In *Black Migration to South Africa: A Selection of Policy-Oriented Research,* ed. J. Bohning. Geneva: International Labour Office.

———. 1981b. "The Impact of Labour Migration in South Africa." *Journal of Development Studies* 17 (3): 59–76.

Gordon, R. 1977. *Mines, Masters, and Migrants.* Johannesburg: Ravan.

Grosz, E. 1995. "Women, Chora, Dwelling." In *Postmodern Cities and Spaces,* ed. S. Watson and K. Gibson, 47–58. Oxford: Blackwell.

Guba, E. 1990. *The Paradigm Dialog.* London: Sage Publications.

Hanks, D., and M. Lipire. 1993. "South African Migration and the Effects on Family." *Marriage and Family Review* 19 (1–2): 175–92.

Harries, P. 1990. "Symbols and Sexuality: Culture and Identity on the Early Witwatersrand Gold Mines." *Gender and History* 2 (3): 318–36.

Harris, V. 1987. "Black-Owned Land, White Farmers, and the State in Northern Natal, 1910–1936." *Journal of Natal and Zulu History* 10:51–76.

Hart, D., and G. Pirie. 1984. "The Sight and Soul of Sophiatown." *Geographical Review* 74:38–47.

Hassim, S. 1993. "Family, Motherhood, and Zulu Nationalism: The Place of the Politics of the Inkatha Women's Brigade." *Feminist Review* 43:1–25.

Hassim, S., and L. Stiebel. 1993. "The Semiotics of Struggle: Gender Representations in the Natal Violence." PRIF Reports, no. 30. Frankfurt: Peace Research Institute Frankfurt.

Heise, L. 1997. "Violence, Sexuality, and Women's Lives." In *The Gender Sexuality Reader: Culture, History, Political Economy,* ed. R. Lancaster and M. Leonardo, 411–33. New York: Routledge.

Hellmann, E. 1935. "Native Life in a Johannesburg Slum Yard." *Africa* 3:34–62.

———. 1948. *Rooiyard, a Sociological Survey of an Urban Native Slum Yard.* Oxford: Oxford University Press.

Heyns, M. 1998. "A Man's World: White South African Gay Writing and the State of Emergency." In *Writing South Africa: Literature, Apartheid, and Democracy, 1970–1995,* ed. D. Attridge and R. Jolly, 108–22. Cambridge: Cambridge University Press.

Hindson, D. 1987. "Urbanization and Influx Control Policy in the 1970s and 1980s: From Territorial Apartheid to Regional Spatial Ordering." In *Pass Controls and the Urban African Proletariat,* ed. D. Hindson, 80–89. Johannesburg: Ravan.

hooks, b. 1991. Yearning: Race, Gender, and Cultural Politics, Boston: South End Press.

Hunt, C. 1989. "Migrant Labour and Sexually Transmitted Diseases: AIDS in Africa." *Journal of Social Behavior* 30 (4): 353–80.

Hyden, G. 1983. *No Short Cuts to Progress: African Development Management in Perspective.* London: Heinemann.

Industrial Monitor. 1993. "ANC/IFP Support in Reef Townships and Hostels." *Indicator SA* 10 (2): 21.

JanMohamed, A. 1992. "Sexuality on/of the Racial Border: Foucault, Wright, and Articulation of 'Racialized Sexuality.'" In *Discourses in Sexuality: From Aristotle to Aids,* ed. D. Stanton, 94–116. Ann Arbor: University of Michigan Press.

Jochelson, K. 1995. "Women, Migrancy, and Movality." *Journal of Southern African Studies* 21 (2): 323–32.

Jochelson, K., M. Mothielei, and J. Leger. 1991. "Human Immunodeficiency Virus and Migrant Labor in South Africa." *Journal of Health Services* 21 (1): 157–73.

Jones, S. 1993. *Assaulting Childhood: Children's Experiences of Migrancy and Hostel Life in South Africa.* Johannesburg: Witwatersrand University Press.

Joubert, E. 1985. *Poppie Nongena.* New York: Norton.

Karim, Q., and S. Karim. 1999. *Epidemiology of HIV in South Africa.* Pretoria: South African Medical Research Council: Center for Epidemiological Research in South Africa, Medical Research Council, Southern African Fogarty HIV/AIDS International Training and Research Program, and the International AIDS Vaccine Initiative.

Keenan, J. 1981. "Migrants Awake: The 1980 Municipal Strike." *South African Labour Review* 7 (7): 4–60.

Kendall, 1998. "'When a Woman Loves a Woman' in Lesotho: Love, Sex, and the (Western) Construction of Homophobia." In *Boy-Wives and Female Husbands: Studies in African Homosexualities,* ed. S. Murray and W. Roscoe, 223–41. New York: St. Martin's Press.

Khosa, M. 1998. "Sisters on the Wheel: Gender Relations in the Taxi Industry in Durban." In *Changing Gender Relations in Southern Africa: Issues of Urban Life,* ed. E. Mapetla, A. Larsson, and A. Schlyter, 77–100. Lesotho: Institute of Southern African Studies.

Kirmani, M., and D. Munyakho. 1996. "The Impact of Structural Adjustment Programs on Women and AIDS." In *Women's Experiences with HIV/AIDS: An International Perspective,* ed. L. Lond and E. Ankrah, 160–78. New York: Columbia University Press.

Klasen, S. 2000. "Measuring Poverty and Deprivation in South Africa." *Review of Income and Wealth* 46 (1): 33–58.

Koch, E. 1981. "Without Visible Means of Subsistence: Slumyard Culture in Johannesburg, 1918–1940." In *Town and Countryside in the Transvaal,* ed. B. Bozzoli, 151–75. Johannesburg: Ravan.

Krog, A. 1998. *Country of My Skull.* Johannesburg: Random House.

Laburn, C., and K. McNamara. 1980. "Black Migrant Workers Contact with Home." *Human Resources Monitoring Report* 4 (5): 1–7.

Lather, P. 1988. "Feminist Perspectives on Empowering Research Methodologies." *Women's Studies International Forum* 11:569–81.

Lefebvre, H. 1991. *The Production of Space.* Oxford: Blackwell.

Leliveld, A. 1997. "The Effects of Restrictive South African Migrant Labor Policy on the Survival of Rural Households in Southern Africa: A Case from Rural Swaziland." *World Development* 25 (11): 1839–49.

Lemon, A. 1982. "Migrant Labour and Frontier Commuters: Reorganizing South Africa's Black Labour Supply." In *Living under Apartheid,* ed. D. Smith, 64–89. London: George Allen and Unwin.

Lipton, M. 1980. "Men of Two Worlds: Migrant Labor in South Africa." *Optima* 29 (2–3): 72–101.

Low, A. 1986. *Agricultural Development in Southern Africa: Farm-Households Economics and the Food Crisis.* London: James Currey.

Mabin, A. 1986. "Labour, Capital, Class Struggle, and the Origins of Residential Segregation in Kimberley, 1880–1920." *Journal of Historical Geography* 12:4–26.

MacDonald, D. 1997. "Neither from Above, Nor Below: Municipal Bureaucrats and Environmental Policy in Cape Town, South Africa." *Canadian Journal of African Studies* 30 (2): 315–40.

Mackay, C. 1999. "Housing Policy in South Africa: The Challenge of Delivery." *Housing Studies* 14 (3): 387–99.

Mager, A., and G. Minkley. 1993. "Reaping the Whirlwind: The East London Riots of 1952." In *Apartheid's Genesis, 1935–1962,* ed. P. Bonner, P. Delius, and D. Posel, 229–51. Johannesburg: Witwatersrand University Press.

Mamdani, M. 1996. *Citizen and Subject: Contemporary Africa and the Legacy of Late Colonialism.* Princeton: Princeton University Press.

Marks, S., and E. Unterhalter. 1978. "Women and the Migrant Labour System in Southern Africa." Paper presented at the Conference on Migratory Labour in Southern Africa, Lusaka, Republic of Zambia, April 4–8.

Mashabela, H. 1988. *Townships of the PWV.* Johannesburg: South African Institute of Race Relations.

Massey, D. 1993. "Power Geometry and a Progressive Sense of Place." In *Mapping the Futures: Local Cultures, Global Change,* ed. J. Bird, B. Curtis, T. Putnam, G. Robertson, and L. Tickner, 59–69. London: Routledge.

Mayer, P. 1961. *Townsmen or Tribesmen: Conservation and the Process of Urbanization in a South African City.* Cape Town: Oxford University Press.

———. 1980. *Black Villagers in an Industrial Society.* Cape Town: Oxford University Press.

Mbeki, T. 1998: *Africa: The Time Has Come.* Cape Town: Tafelberg Publishers, Ltd.

McClintock, A. 1995. *Imperial Leather: Race, Gender, and Sexuality in the Colonial Contest.* New York: Routledge.

McFadden, P. 1992. "Sex, Sexuality, and the Problems of AIDS in Africa." In *Gender in Southern Africa: Conceptual and Theoretical Issues*, ed. R. Meena, 157–95. Harare: SAPES.

Michie, J., and V. Padayachee. 1997. *The Political Economy of South Africa's Transition: Policy Perspectives in the Late 1990's*. London: Dryden.

Miles, M. 1993. "Missing Women: Reflections on the Experiences of Swazi Migrant Women on the Rand, 1920–1970." *GeoJournal* 30 (1): 85–91.

Miles, M., and J. Crush. 1993. "Personal Narratives as Interactive Texts: Collecting and Interpreting Migrant Life-Histories." *Professional Geographer* 45 (1): 87–94.

Minnaar, A. 1989. "The South African Maize Industry's Response to the Great Depression and the Beginnings of Large-Scale State Intervention, 1929–1934." *South African Journal of Economic History* 4 (1): 68–78.

———, ed. 1993. *Communities in Isolation: Perspectives on Hostels in South Africa*. Goldstone Hostels Report 1993. Pretoria: Human Sciences Research Council.

Mohlabe, H. 1970. "Moral Effects of the System of Migratory Labour on the Labourer and His Family." Paper presented to the Consultation on Migrant Labour and Church Involvement, Natal, August.

Moodie, T. 1980. "The Formal and Informal Social Structure of a South African Gold Mine." *Human Relations* 33:555–74.

———. 1988. "Migrancy and Male Sexuality on the South African Gold Mines." *Journal of Southern African Studies* 14 (2): 228–56.

———. 1992. "Town Women and Country Wives: Migrant Labour, Family Politics, and Housing Preferences at Vaal Reefs." *Labour, Capital, and Society* 25 (1): 116–32.

——— (with V. Ndatshe). 1994. *Going for Gold: Men, Mines, and Migration*. Berkeley: University of California Press.

Moroney, S. 1978. "The Development of the Compound as a Mechanism of Worker Control, 1900–1912." *South African Labour Bulletin* 4 (3): 29–49.

Murray, C. 1981. "Migrant Labour and Changing Family Structure in the Rural Periphery of South Africa." *Journal of Southern African Studies* 6 (2): 139–56.

Naanen, B. 1991. "Itinerant Gold Mines: Prostitution in the Cross River Basin of Nigeria, 1930–1950." *African Studies Review* 34 (2): 57–79.

Nast, H., and M. Wilson. 1994. "Lawful Transgressions: This Is the House That Jackie Built . . ." *Assemblage* 24:49–55.

Nelson, J. 1976. "Sojourners versus New Urbanites: Causes and Consequences of Temporary versus Permanent Migration." *Economic Development and Cultural Change* 24:721–57.

O'Brien, D. 1977. "Female Husbands in Southern Bantu Societies." In *Sexual Stratification: A Cross-Cultural View,* ed. A. Schlegel, 109–26. New York: Columbia University Press.

Olivier, J. 1993. Preface to *Communities in Isolation: Perspectives on Hostels in South Africa.* Goldstone Hostels Report 1993, ed. A. Minnaar, i. Pretoria: Human Sciences Research Council.

O'Meara, D. 1996. *Forty Lost Years: The Apartheid State and the Politics of the National Party, 1948–1994.* Athens: Ohio University Press.

Parpart, J. 1986. "Class and Gender on the Copperbelt: Women in Northern Rhodesian Copper Mining Communities, 1926–1964." In *Women and Class In Africa,* ed. C. Robertson and I. Berger, 60–81. New York: Cambridge University Press.

Paton, A. 1950. *Cry, the Beloved Country.* New York: Scribner's.

Patton, C. 1992. "From Nation to Family: Containing 'African AIDS.'" In *Nationalisms and Sexualities,* ed. A. Parker, M. Russo, D. Sommer, and P. Yaeger, 218–34. New York: Routledge.

Payze, C., and T. Keith. 1993. "Everyday Life in South African Hostels." In *Communities in Isolation: Perspectives on Hostels in South Africa.* Goldstone Hostels Report 1993, ed. A. Minnaar, 48–63. Pretoria: Human Sciences Research Council.

Pikholz, L. 1997. "Managing Politics and Storytelling: Meeting the Challenge of Upgrading Informal Housing in South Africa." *Habitat International* 21 (4): 377–82.

Pinnock, D. 1981. *TELONA: Some Reflections of the Work of a Private Labour Recruiter.* Southern Africa Labour and Development Research Unit Working Paper no. 31. Cape Town: University of Cape Town.

Pirie, G. 1991. "Kimberley." In *Homes Apart: South Africa's Segregated Cities,* ed. A. Lemon, 120–28. Cape Town: David Philip.

Pirie, G., and M. da Silva. 1986. "Hostels for African Migrants in Greater Johannesburg." *GeoJournal* 12:173–82.

Platzky, L., and C. Walker. 1985. *The Surplus People: Forced Removals in South Africa.* Johannesburg: Ravan.

Posel, D. 1991. *The Making of Apartheid, 1948–1961: Conflict and Compromise.* Oxford: Clarendon Press.

Ramphele, M. 1986. "The Male and Female Dynamics amongst Migrant Workers in the Western Cape." *Social Dynamics* 12 (1): 15–25.

———. 1989a. "The Dynamics of Gender Politics in the Hostels of Cape Town: Another Legacy of the South African Migrant Labour System." *Journal of Southern African Studies* 15:393–414.

———. 1989b. "Empowerment and the Politics of Space." Rama Mehta Lecture, Bunting Institute, Radcliffe College, Harvard University.

————. 1993. *A Bed Called Home: Life in the Migrant Labour Hostels of Cape Town*. Cape Town: David Philip.

Rao Gupta, G. 1993. "Women and HIV: Lessons from a Multicountry Research Project." Paper presented at the Working Group on Sexual Behaviour Research Conference: International Perspectives in Sex Research, Rio de Janeiro, April 22–25.

Reed, D. 1994. *Beloved Country: South Africa's Silent Wars*. Johannesburg: Jonathan Ball Publishers.

Reynolds, P. 1988. *Men without Children*. Cape Town: University of Cape Town.

Rich, A. 1993. "Compulsory Heterosexuality and Lesbian Existence." In *The Lesbian and Gay Studies Reader*, ed. H. Abelove, M. Barale, and D. Halperin, 227–54. New York: Routledge.

Robertson, M., and J. McCarthy. 1988. "'Orderly Urbanization': The New Influx Control." *Natal University Law and Society Review* 2:155–74.

Robinson, J. 1992. "Abandoning Androcentrism? A Future for Gender Studies in South African Geography." In *Geography in a Changing South Africa*, ed. C. Rogerson and J. McCarthy, 123–37. Cape Town: Oxford University Press.

————. 1996. *The Power of Apartheid: State, Power, and Space in South African Cities*. Oxford: Butterworth-Heinemann.

Rosen-Prinz, B., and F. Prinz. 1978. *Migrant Labour and Rural Homesteads: An Investigation into the Sociological Dimensions of the Migrant Labour System in Swaziland*. World Employment Program Working Paper, International Labour Organization.

Rubenstein, S. 1993. "The Story of a Hostel Project: Vosloorus Nguni Hostel." In *Communities in Isolation: Perspectives on Hostels in South Africa*. Goldstone Hostels Report 1993, ed. A. Minnaar, 143–55. Pretoria: Human Sciences Research Council.

Rubin, G. 1984. "Thinking Sex: Notes for a Radical Theory of the Politics of Sexuality." In *Pleasure and Danger: Exploring Female Sexuality*, ed. C. Vance. Boston: Routledge and Kegan Paul.

Russell, M. 1983. "Boundaries and Structures in the Swaziland Homestead." Research Paper no. 8, Social Science Research Unit, University of Swaziland, Kwaluseni.

————. 1993. "Are Households Universal? Of Misunderstanding Domestic Groups in Swaziland." *Development and Change* 24 (4): 55–87.

Said, E. 1993. *Culture and Imperialism*. New York: Vintage Books.

SAIRR (South African Institute of Race Relations). 1997. *South Africa Survey, 1996/97*. Johannesburg: South African Institute of Race Relations.

————. 1998. *South Africa Survey, 1997/98*. Johannesburg: South African Institute of Race Relations.

Sansom, B. 1974. "Traditional Economic Systems." In *The Bantu-Speaking Peoples of Southern Africa,* ed. W. Hammond-Tooke, 135–76. London: Routledge and Kegan Paul.

Schapera, I. 1947. *Migrant Labor and Tribal Life: A Study of Conditions.* London: Oxford University Press.

Schlyter, A. 1996. *A Place to Live: Gender Research on Housing in Africa.* Uppsala: Nordiska Afrikainstitutet.

Schmidt, E. 1991. "Patriarchy, Capitalism, and the Colonial State in Zimbabwe." *Signs* 16 (4): 732–56.

Schreiner, G. 1991. "Transforming Hostels." *Indicator SA* 8 (3): 87–88.

Segal, L. 1991. "The Human Face." *Journal of Southern African Studies* 18 (1): 190–231.

Sen, A. 1999. *Development as Freedom.* New York: Anchor Books.

Sharp, J., and J. Spiegel. 1990. "Women and Wages: Gender and the Control of Income in Farm and Bantustan Homelands." *Journal of Southern African Studies* 16 (3): 527–49.

Shaw, M. 1993. "Hostels, Violence, and the Possibility of Lasting Peace: A Case Study of Ratanda Township, Heidelberg." In *Communities in Isolation: Perspectives on Hostels in South Africa.* Goldstone Hostels Report 1993, ed. A. Minnaar, 156–68. Pretoria: Human Sciences Research Council.

Sher, R., E. Antimes, B. Reid, and H. Patel. 1981. *HIV Antibody Prevalence in Black Miners between 1970 and 1974.* Johannesburg: Witwatersrand University Press.

Sherman, J. 2000. "Serving the Natives: Whiteness as the Price of Hospitality in South African Yiddish Literature." *Journal of Southern African Studies* 26 (3): 505–21.

Sinclair, M. 1998. "Community, Identity, and Gender in Migrant Societies of Southern Africa: Emerging Epistemological Challenges." *International Affairs* 74 (2): 339–53.

Singh, A. 1999. "Women and Empowerment through the 'Economy of Affection' in KwaZulu-Natal: Its Significance for Sustainable Development." *Development Southern Africa* 16 (3): 467–88.

Sitas, A. 1985. "Moral Formation and Struggles amongst Migrant Workers on the East Rand." *Laubour, Capital, Society* 18 (2): 372–401.

———. 1996. "The New Tribalism: Hostels and Violence." *Journal of Southern African Studies* 22 (2): 235–48.

Spivak, G. 1987. *In Other Worlds: Essays in Cultural Politics.* New York: Routledge.

Smit, D., and V. Vedalankar. 1993. "National Agreement Must Be Translated Locally." *Reconstruct: A Work in Progress Supplement* 12:2–3.

Smith, D. 1992. *The Apartheid City and Beyond: Urbanization and Social Change in South Africa.* London: Routledge.

South Africa. 1934. *Hansard Parliamentary Debates.* Cape Town: Government Printers.

———. 1936. *Hansard Parliamentary Debates.* Cape Town: Government Printers.

———. 1990. *South African Census.* Cape Town: Government Printers.

———. 1991. *Goldstone Commission of Inquiry into Hostel Violence.* Cape Town: Government Printers.

———. 1994. *Government Gazette* 343 (15466). Cape Town: Government Printer.

———. 1996. *South African Census.* <http://www.statssa.gov.za/>.

———. 1998. *Truth and Reconciliation Commission: Final Report.* 5 vols. <http://www.polity.org.za/govdocs/commissions/1998/trc/index.htm>.

SARB (South African Reserve Bank). 1991. *Annual Review.* Pretoria: Government Printers.

Spiegel, A. 1991. "Polygyny as Myth: Towards Understanding Extramarital Relations in Lesotho." In *Tradition and Transition in Southern Africa (Festschrift for Philip and Iona Mayer),* ed. A. Spiegel and P. McAllister, 145–66. Johannesburg: Witwatersrand University Press.

Stubbs, J. 1984. "Some Thoughts on the Life Story Method in Labour History and Research on Rural Women." *Institute of Development Studies Bulletin* 15:34–37.

Swanson, M. 1977. "The Sanitation Syndrome: Bubonic Plague and Urban Native Policy in the Cape Colony, 1900–1909." *Journal of African History* 18:387–410.

Taylor, J. 1990. "The Reorganization of Mine Labour Recruitment in Southern Africa: Evidence from Botswana." *International Migration Review* 24:250–72.

Tepperman, J. D. 2002. "Truth and Consequences." *Foreign Affairs,* March–April, 128–45.

Tinker, I., and G. Summerfield. 1999. *Women's Rights to House and Land: China, Laos, Vietnam.* Boulder: Lynne Rienner Publishers.

Tomlinson, R. 1994. *Urban Development Planning: Lessons for the Economic Reconstruction of South Africa's Cities.* London: Zed Books.

Turrell, R. 1984. "Kimberley's Model Compounds." *Journal of African History* 25:59–76.

Valodia, I. 1998. "Finance, State Expenditure, S.A. Revenue Service, and Central Statistical Service." In *The Third Women's Budget,* ed. D. Budlender. Cape Town: Idasa.

van der Vliet, V. 1991. "Traditional Husbands, Modern Wives? Constructing Marriages in a South African Township." *African Studies* 50:219–41.

van Onselen, C. 1996. *The Seed Is Mine: The Life of Kas Maine, a South African Sharecropper, 1894-1985.* Cape Town: David Phillip.

Waetjen, T. 1999. "The 'Home' in Homeland: Gender, National Space, and Inkatha's Politics of Ethnicity." *Ethnic and Racial Studies* 22 (4): 653–78.

Walker, C. 1991. "Gender and the Development of the Migrant Labour System, c. 1850–1930: An Overview." In *Women and Gender in Southern Africa to 1945,* ed. C. Walker, 168–96. Cape Town: David Philip.

———. 1992. Book review of *Women of Phokeng* by B. Bozzoli. *Social Dynamics* 18 (2) 75–77.

Webster, D. 1991. "Abafazi Bathonga Bafihlakala: Ethnicity and Gender in a KwaZulu Border Community." In *Tradition and Transition in Southern Africa (Festschrift for Philip and Iona Mayer),* ed. A. Spiegel and P. McAllister, 243–71. Johannesburg: Witwatersrand University Press.

Wells, J. 1993. *We Now Demand!: The History of Women's Resistance to Pass Laws in South Africa.* Johannesburg: Witwatersrand University Press.

Weisman, L. 1994. *Discrimination by Design: A Feminist Critique of the Man-Made Environment.* Urbana: University of Illinois Press.

Wentzel, M. 1993. "Historical Origins of Hostels in South Africa: Migrant Labour and Compounds." In *Communities in Isolation: Perspectives on Hostels in South Africa.* Goldstone Hostels Report 1993, ed. A. Minnaar, 1–9. Pretoria: Human Sciences Research Council.

West, C. 1994. *Race Matters.* New York: Vintage Books.

White, L. 1990. *The Comforts of Home: Prostitution in Colonial Nairobi.* Chicago: University of Chicago Press.

Wilson, F. 1972. *Migrant Labour: Report to the South African Council of Churches.* Johannesburg: South African Council of Churches/SPRO-CAS.

Wilson, F., and M. Ramphele. 1989. *Uprooting Poverty: The South African Challenge.* Cape Town: David Philip.

Zulu, P. 1993. "Hostels in the Greater Durban Area: A Case Study of the Kwa-Mashu and Umlazi Hostels." In *Communities in Isolation: Perspectives on Hostels in South Africa,* ed. A. Minnaar, 80–96. Pretoria: Human Sciences Research Council.

INDEX